Study Guide to Accompany
Radiographic Imaging

Study Guide to Accompany
Radiographic Imaging

Mosby's Radiographic Instructional Series

with illustrations

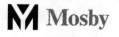 Mosby

St. Louis Baltimore Boston Carlsbad Chicago Naples New York Philadelphia Portland
London Madrid Mexico City Singapore Sydney Tokyo Toronto Wiesbaden

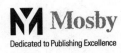
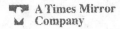

Executive Editor: Jeanne Rowland
Developmental Editor: Carole Glauser
Director, Media Production: Theresa Fuchs
Project Manager: Gayle May Morris
Associate Production Editor: Lisa M. Kearney
Manufacturing Manager: Betty Mueller

Printed in the United States of America
Editorial services provided by Tom Lochhaas
Composition by Black Dot

Mosby-Year Book, Inc.
11830 Westline Industrial Drive
St. Louis, MO 63146

ISBN 0-8151-5408-9

98 99 00 01 02 / 9 8 7 6 5 4 3 2 1

Introduction

Radiographic Imaging Study Guide is designed to accompany the Radiographic Imaging multimedia program in *Mosby's Radiographic Instructional Series*. This study guide can be used with either the slide/audiotape or the CD-ROM version of the program. The multimedia portion of this instructional program, along with the study guide, will provide a solid foundation in the principles of radiographic imaging such as equipment components, factors affecting recorded detail, technique, and film processing, and how these principles can be applied in the clinical setting. The program can be used for both instruction and review.

The eight modules in this study guide correspond to the eight modules of the multimedia program. Usually you will find it more effective to experience the multimedia program first and then read and work through the accompanying module in the study guide. The different parts of each module in the study guide allow you to review and apply what you learn from the multimedia module as much or as little as you find helpful. Answers to the various exercises appear at the end of each module in the study guide.

Self-Assessment Pretest is a group of 10 multiple-choice questions designed to help you determine how much of the module's material you have already mastered from the multimedia program before beginning to review this material in the study guide. If you incorrectly answered some questions, pay more attention to those subjects as you proceed through the other parts of the study guide.

Key Terms is a brief glossary section that defines important terms introduced in the multimedia module. It is important to gain a clear understanding of these terms and the concepts they represent before proceeding. Take a moment to read quickly through these definitions, and when you encounter items with which you are not yet comfortable, give special attention to their meaning. These terms will continue to be used in following parts, helping you become more familiar with them and their importance in radiography.

Topical Outline presents in a brief format the primary information and knowledge covered by the multimedia module. As when reading the key terms definitions, pay particular attention to areas you are not confident you understand.

Review gives you a chance to interact with the material that has been briefly introduced through the Key Terms and Topical Outline sections. You are encouraged to write in the terms and phrases indicated by the blank lines in these descriptive and explanatory statements. Do not view this as a test. What is important in this exercise is that you are becoming more familiar with the terminology and concepts related to the module's content. Some artwork is included in this section, usually a variation of illustrations used in the multimedia program, to enhance the learning and retention of important concepts or processes.

Learning Quiz is unique among the various parts in that it is not intended to be used by those who have worked through the CD-ROM version of the multimedia program in what is called the interactive "student mode"—a student at the computer individually working through the learning program. In other words, you will want to complete this section if you viewed the slide/audio version or the CD-ROM program in "instructor" mode, without experiencing the program individually at the computer. If you have already worked through the full interactive program at the computer, you can, if you choose, skip over this section, which includes exercises you will already have experienced in the computer tutorial. On the other hand, repeating these exercises in the study guide format may be valuable as additional review. These exercises are designed to help you increase your mastery of the material by answering questions that require knowledge and understanding of key information that has been presented so far.

Applications addresses the module's concepts and information at a higher level by asking questions that require you to apply what you have learned in different situations or examples. This necessitates a fuller understanding of the material—how the principles of physics apply to the specific topic. These questions are in some ways the most *difficult* in the module because they involve more than just defining terms or repeating information. Take your time with these. If you have difficulty, return to the Key Terms and Outline to review. If you do well in answering these questions, you probably have a good grasp of the material in this module.

Posttest is the final section in each module in the study guide. It consists of an average of 20 multiple-choice questions designed to assess your understanding and retention of the information in the module after having worked through the preceding study guide sections. The answers to this section, unlike other sections, are not included in this study guide but are printed in the instructor's manual for the program—this is to allow your course instructor to use the posttest for more formal evaluation if desired.

This study guide is intended to make your learning experience more satisfying, while at the same time helping you learn, master, and remember what may be new or difficult material. The authors hope you find it an enjoyable experience.

Contents

Study Guide to Accompany
Radiographic Imaging

Radiographic Equipment

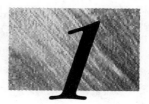

Self-Assessment Pretest

Use this pretest to assess your knowledge of the material in this module before you begin to work through the following exercises. Circle the best answer for each of the following questions. The answers are at the end of this module.

1. What first alerted early researchers to the potential dangers of x-ray beams?
   a. Radiation burns on the skin of those heavily exposed
   b. Nausea and vomiting by those being radiographed
   c. The use of Geiger counters
   d. A higher incidence of cancers in those exposed

2. One of the first, and still most important, uses of computed tomography is to obtain images of which of the following?
   a. Muscles
   b. Gastrointestinal motility
   c. The brain
   d. Contrast media

3. The primary difference between radiography and fluoroscopy is the difference between which of the following?
   a. Cathodes and anodes
   b. High kVp and low kVp
   c. X-rays and gamma rays
   d. Static and dynamic images

4. Which of the following is an example of a dedicated radiographic unit?
   a. Mammography unit
   b. Head unit
   c. Chest unit
   d. All of the above
   e. None of the above

5. Which of these imaging modalities can be used in mobile units?
   a. Radiography and fluoroscopy
   b. Radiography and computed tomography
   c. Radiography, fluoroscopy, and computed tomography
   d. Radiography only

6. What is the purpose of a grid?
   a. To help position the patient more exactly
   b. To absorb scatter radiation before it reaches the film
   c. To hold the radiographic film in place during the exposure
   d. To amplify the x-ray beam

7. In linear tomography, which of the following is true?
   a. The film and x-ray tube both move during the exposure.
   b. The film moves while the tube remains fixed.
   c. The tube moves while the film remains fixed.
   d. The image is generated by a computer.

8. Computed tomography does which of the following?
   a. Exposes patients to higher doses of radiation
   b. Exposes patients to lower doses of radiation
   c. Exposes patients to the same doses of radiation
   d. Exposes patients to equivalent doses but different kinds of radiation

9. What is the main purpose for the x-ray tube housing?
   a. To cool the x-ray tube
   b. To prevent the x-ray tube from breaking when moved
   c. To focus the x-ray beam the same way a camera lens focuses
   d. To absorb x-rays not included in the primary beam

10. Tube suspension systems include which of the following?
    a. C-arm units
    b. Overhead systems
    c. Floor-to-ceiling systems
    d. All of the above
    e. None of the above

Key Terms

Before continuing, be sure you can define the following key terms.

Bucky assembly: A device invented by the radiographer Gustav Bucky that holds the film and grid and attaches under the radiographic examination table.

C-arm unit: A type of tube suspension system, commonly found in mobile and other equipment, in which the x-ray tube is mounted at one end of the C-arm and the image receptor at the other end.

Cathode ray: A historic term for the flow of electrons from the cathode to the anode in a tube.

Contrast medium: A radiopaque or radiolucent substance injected or ingested into the body for improved visualization of structures in a radiographic or fluoroscopic examination.

Computed tomography: An imaging modality in which a computer creates a cross-sectional image from exposures taken in a complete circle around the body.

Control console: That part of the radiographic equipment where the radiologic technologist sets tube current, voltage, and exposure variables.

Crookes tube: The name for the original glass tube with cathode and anode, named for the nineteenth century scientist William Crookes; the discovery of x-rays was made with a Crookes tube.

Floating table top: A type of table for an imaging examination that allows movement of the surface in all directions in the horizontal plane.

Fluoroscopy: An imaging modality that creates dynamic images on a monitor, generated by x- rays transmitted to an electronic image receptor rather than film.

Grid: A device designed to allow x-rays to be transmitted directly through the patient to the film but to absorb x-rays scattered within the patient before they reach the film.

Head unit: A dedicated radiographic unit with a fixed tube-image receptor arrangement that can be positioned at different angles around the patient's head.

Housing: The part of the x-ray tube assembly that encloses the x-ray tube and functions to cool the tube and to absorb scatter and leakage radiation.

Linear tomography: Also called conventional tomography, this is a system in which the film and x-ray tube are moved in opposite directions during the exposure to blur out structures not in the desired focal plane.

Mammography unit: A dedicated radiographic unit specially designed for breast imaging.

Primary radiation: The radiation in the useful beam from the x-ray tube.

Radiation protection: A general term for protective shielding, equipment, and devices that prevent radiation from reaching the radiographer or the patient except for the desired primary beam.

Radiolucent: Allowing x-rays to pass through without absorption or attenuation; the tabletop, the patient's clothing, etc. should be radiolucent.

Scatter radiation: X-rays produced inside the patient's body or another substance when x-ray photons within the primary beam interact with atoms in that substance to produce Compton or classical scattering of x-ray photons in different directions.

Secondary radiation: Any radiation other than the primary radiation of the useful beam; includes scatter radiation and any leakage radiation from the x-ray tube.

Suspension system: The structural support parts of radiographic equipment that suspend the x-ray tube and allow it to be moved and directed at various angles.

Upright unit: A radiographic unit designed to make radiographic images with the patient standing in front of the image receptor, commonly used for chest radiographs.

Topical Outline

The following material is covered in this module.

I. X-ray beams were discovered in the late nineteenth century and became the focus of much experimentation for decades.
    A. In 1895 Dr. Roentgen discovered that unknown, invisible rays produced by a Crookes tube could pass through objects and make a fluorescent tube glow.
        1. Roentgen discovered that some objects are radiolucent and others radiopaque.

2. By chance Roentgen discovered he could obtain an image of bones within the body by passing x-ray beams through his hand. A radiograph of his wife's hand was the first published radiograph.
B. In 1896 the first medical use was made of radiography to view a broken wrist.
C. In 1898 Dr. Rollins first published warnings of the potential harmful effects of radiation after experiencing skin burns from his experiments with x-ray beams.
D. In the 1940s and 1950s the hazards of x-ray beams were more carefully examined, leading to an increasing interest in protective devices.
E. Now, some 200 million medical and 100 million dental radiographs are made every year in the United States.
F. In the middle and late twentieth century, imaging technology has continued to expand and now includes computed tomography, magnetic resonance imaging, and other diagnostic modalities for imaging body structures. Radiation is also used in the treatment of some conditions such as tumors.

II. Modern radiography has evolved into a wide spectrum of imaging procedures using a variety of types of equipment.
A. Radiography and fluoroscopy are the two main types of radiologic examinations.
1. Radiography uses x-ray beams to produce static images on film.
2. Fluoroscopy uses x-ray beams to produce dynamic images on a monitor.
3. Specialized examinations are used to image different structures and to observe changes within the body such as with the insertion of a catheter or the movement of a fluid through vessels.
B. There are many types of radiographic equipment.
1. Dedicated radiographic equipment is used only for specific functions, such as a head unit or mammography unit.
2. Multipurpose radiographic equipment is used for many different types of examinations.
3. Mobile radiographic or fluoroscopic units are used outside the radiology department, often in emergency rooms, intensive care units, or surgical suites.
C. Examination tables, like the x-ray tube itself, can be angled and moved in various ways to allow very controlled exposure of the desired body area.
D. In addition to the tube and the table, the third key element in all radiographic equipment is the image receptor device, such as the film cassette or the Bucky tray that holds the film and grid, which is usually mounted under the examining table.
E. The fourth key element is the control or operating console, which contains the controls the radiologic technologist uses to set the tube current, voltage, exposure, and other settings for an examination.
F. Conventional tomography and computed tomography are additional modalities using x-ray beams.
1. Conventional, or linear, tomography uses special equipment that moves the film and x-ray tube to produce images that highlight structures in a certain focal plane.
2. In computed tomography, also called CT scanning, a computer creates a cross-sectional image from exposures taken in a complete circle around the body.

III. In addition to the x-ray tube and image receptor, other parts of radiographic equipment are important.
A. The tube housing absorbs x-ray beams that otherwise would "leak" out from the tube in directions other than in the useful beam.
B. The x-ray tube and tube housing are structurally supported, or suspended, in different ways in different types of equipment.
1. An overhead suspension system is mounted on the ceiling, with rails and adjustments to allow the tube to be directed in many different ways.

2. A floor-to-ceiling suspension system mounts the tube on rails mounted to both ceiling and floor.
3. A floor-mounted suspension system uses rails or support columns mounted on the floor or the table.
4. A variety of mobile systems have been developed in which the tube is suspended from a stand on a mobile base.
5. The C-arm suspension system holds the tube on one end of the arm and the image receptor on the other; these systems may be mobile or fixed.

IV. Modern radiology suites generally have permanently installed equipment in a design that also incorporates radiation protection devices.
   A. Lead sheets are often built into the walls of examination rooms to prevent exposure by scatter or leakage radiation.
   B. Secondary radiation protective barriers and shields include a variety of devices to absorb secondary radiation and protect both the radiographer and patient from unwanted exposure.

Review

1. Experimenting with a(n) _____ tube, Dr. Roentgen discovered x-rays when invisible rays made a nearby fluorescent screen _____ .

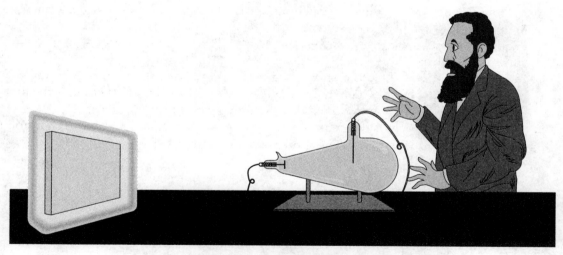

DR. ROENTGEN DISCOVERS X-RAYS IN LAB

2. The stream of _____ passing inside a Crookes tube was formerly called a cathode ray because the electrons flowed from the _____ to the _____.

3. Dr. Rollins became alarmed at the possible harmful effects of _____ after receiving

 burns on his _____ caused by experiments.

4. A treatment use of x-rays, called _____ _____, is used to shrink

 _____.

5. The two basic types of examination procedures using x-rays are called _____

 and _____.

6. Fluoroscopy is different from _____ in that it shows _____

 images on a(n) _____ instead of static images on _____.

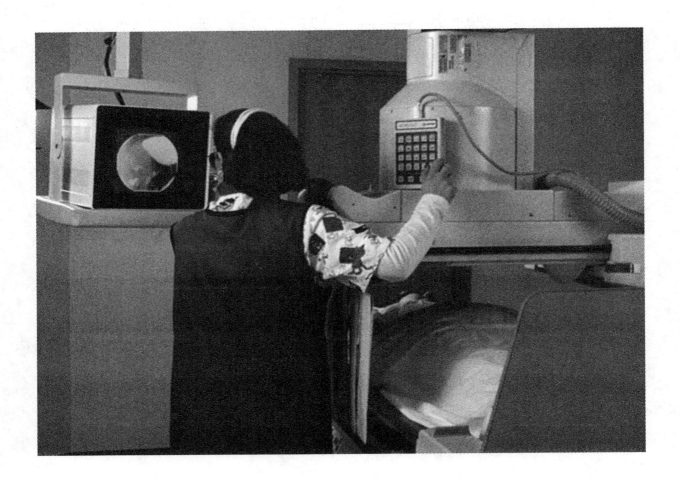

7. The main parts of a radiographic system include the x-ray _____ suspended over the

_____ table and the _____ tray or assembly that holds the

film and _____.

8. An examination table should be _____ and easy to _____.

9. Grids are used to absorb _____ radiation, caused when x-ray _____

interact within the patient and cause _____ to be emitted at other angles.

10. Special radiographic units such as mammographic units are called _____, as

opposed to general equipment that can be used for a variety of types of examinations. Other

examples include _____ units and _____units.

11. In conventional, or _____ , tomography the film and _____

move in opposite directions to blur out structures not in the desired

_____.

12. CT, the abbreviation for _____ _____, creates cross-sec-

tional _____ assembled by a(n) _____ as the x-ray tube and

image receptor rotate in a full _____ around the patient.

13. _____ is used to observe the movement of something inside the body,

such as a(n) _____ _____ that is ingested and moves through

the gastrointestinal system.

14. The x-ray tube _____ absorbs x-rays except those in the _____,

or useful, beam. This helps prevent _____ radiation from reaching the

patient or radiographer.

15. Permanently installed radiographic equipment may include a variety of _____ systems for holding the x-ray tube. Different kinds of examination _____ also allow tilting and movement in side-to-side directions.

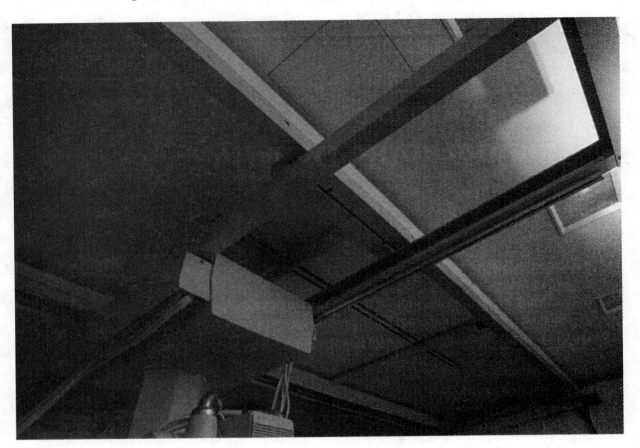

16. A C-arm system has the _____ at one end of the arm and the _____ at the other end.

17. Mobile radiographic units are commonly used in _____ and _____.

18. _____ is often built into the walls of radiographic examination rooms to absorb radiation. _____ barriers are another kind of device used to shield radiographers and others from secondary radiation.

Learning Quiz

The following material includes interactive exercises found in the CD-ROM version of this module operated in the "Student Mode." These questions will allow you to review the concepts presented in this module and will help you gain a more complete understanding of the material.

1. What elements were inside the early Crookes tubes with which Dr. Roentgen discovered x-rays?

2. In the early days, right after the discovery of x-rays, how were x-rays first used?

3. At the turn of the century, x-rays were being widely used in many ways, often with virtually no protection. When were the harmful effects discovered?

4. What is an R/F unit, and what is it used for?

5. Even with fixed radiographic equipment, some parts of the equipment can be physically manipulated to get better images. What parts can be moved and in what ways?

6. What kinds of exams are usually done with the patient standing up, rather than lying on the table?

7. Describe at least three functions of the x-ray tube housing.

8. Marie Curie was one of the first to use mobile radiographic units. How?

9. What is the difference between primary and secondary radiation? Why is protection needed from both?

Applications

1. Name as many common applications for CT scanning as you can think of.

2. Explain the fundamental difference between radiography and fluoroscopy. Give one or more examples of the applications of each.

3. Describe the characteristics of the ideal examination table. For each characteristic you list, explain its benefit.

4. Describe the three main parts of a radiographic equipment system.

5. Explain what is unique about a radiographic unit dedicated for mammography.

6. Name one of the most common procedures in which a contrast medium is injected into the body. What is it used to evaluate?

7. List three or more places where mobile radiographic equipment is often used.

8. Name as many types of common protective devices that help shield the radiographer from radiation during examinations.

Posttest

Circle the best answer for each of the following questions. Your instructor has the correct answers.

1. What was the earliest tube used in the discovery of x-rays called?
   a. Roentgen tube
   b. Crookes tube
   c. Rollins tube
   d. Sodium vapor tube

2. About how many medical and dental radiographs are taken every year in the United States?
   a. 1 million
   b. 50 million
   c. 300 million
   d. 2 billion

3. Radiography, computed tomography, ultrasonography, and MRI are similar in that all involve which of the following?
   a. X-radiation passing through the body
   b. Electromagnetic energy passing through the body
   c. Imaging structures inside the body
   d. None of the above

4. What is a common use of fluoroscopy?
   a. To track the insertion of a catheter
   b. To observe a fluid moving through the gastrointestinal tract
   c. To see the movement of a contrast medium in blood vessels
   d. All of the above
   e. None of the above

5. Dynamic fluoroscopic images are shown on which of the following?
   a. A monitor
   b. Fluoroscopic film
   c. Both a monitor and fluoroscopic film
   d. Standard radiographic film

6. What does a floating radiographic table do?
   a. Floats over a shallow pool of water
   b. Moves laterally but not longitudinally
   c. Moves longitudinally but not laterally
   d. Moves both laterally and longitudinally

7. What must the standard radiographic tabletop always be?
   a. Radiolucent
   b. Radiopaque
   c. Shielded from the primary beam
   d. All of the above

8. What is the source of most of the scatter radiation that grids are designed to absorb?
   a. The Bucky assembly
   b. The x-ray tube housing
   c. The radiographic film
   d. The patient

9. Why is a barrier positioned between the patient area and the operating console?
   a. To prevent the patient from seeing the controls and settings
   b. To prevent radiation from reaching the radiographer
   c. To protect delicate electronic equipment from x-ray damage
   d. To prevent scatter radiation from the console from reaching the film

10. On what principle does linear tomography work?
    a. Alpha and gamma rays react in special ways to create a different image.
    b. Averaging multiple exposures produces a clearer image than any one exposure.
    c. By moving the x-ray tube and film in opposite directions, only structures in a certain focal plane are in focus.
    d. The computer can assemble a cross-sectional image from multiple exposures.

11. In computed tomography, how does the x-ray tube move?
    a. In a full circle around the patient
    b. Back and forth in a half-circle under and around the patient
    c. Side-to-side in a horizontal plane over the patient
    d. None of the above

12. Without a housing around the x-ray tube, which of the following would be true?
    a. No x-rays could reach the patient.
    b. The x-ray tube would rapidly overheat.
    c. The x-ray tube would be easily broken when moved.
    d. X-rays would emerge in all directions from the tube.

13. Which of the following is true of a tube suspension system?
    a. It supports the x-ray tube.
    b. It may be fixed or mobile.
    c. It allows movement of the x-ray tube.
    d. All of the above
    e. None of the above

14. In a C-arm suspension system, you can adjust which of the following?
    a. The distance between the tube and the image receptor
    b. The angle of the C-arm
    c. Both of the above
    d. Neither of the above

15. Locks on an overhead tube suspension system prevent which of the following?
    a. Theft
    b. Electrical shock
    c. Unwanted movement of the equipment
    d. All of the above

16. A mobile radiographic unit may be used in which of the following?
    a. An emergency room
    b. An operating room
    c. An intensive care unit
    d. All of the above
    e. None of the above

17. Which of the following is a challenge in using mobile radiographic equipment?
    a. Positioning very ill patients
    b. Moving the heavy equipment
    c. Arranging for necessary electrical power levels outside the radiology department
    d. All of the above
    e. None of the above

18. Radiation protection built into the radiology department may include which of the following?
    a. Thick aluminum walls
    b. Flowing water absorption systems
    c. Sheets of lead built into the walls
    d. All of the above
    e. None of the above

19. Protection from scatter radiation includes which of the following?
    a. X-ray tube housing
    b. The radiographic tabletop
    c. Barriers between the radiographer and the patient
    d. All of the above
    e. None of the above

20. Materials that may be used in secondary radiation barriers include which of the following?
    a. Glass
    b. Lead acrylic
    c. Gypsum board
    d. All of the above
    e. None of the above

Answer Key

Answers to Pretest

1. a

2. c

3. d

4. d

5. a

6. b

7. a

8. a

9. d

10. d

Answers to Review

1. Crookes, glow

2. Electrons, cathode, anode

3. X-rays, hand

4. Radiation therapy, tumors

5. Radiography, fluoroscopy

6. Radiography, dynamic, monitor, film

7. Tube, examination, Bucky, grid

8. Radiolucent, clean

9. Scatter, photons, x-rays (or photons)

10. Dedicated, head, chest (or upright)

11. Linear, x-ray tube, focal plane

12. Computed tomography, images, computer, circle

13. Fluoroscopy, contrast medium

14. Housing, primary, leakage (or secondary)

15. Suspension, tables

16. X-ray tube, image receptor

17. Emergency rooms, intensive care units (or patient rooms)

18. Lead, protective

Answers to Learning Quiz

1. The early Crookes tube had a simple design, with positive and negative electrodes in a sealed glass tube. The air was pumped out, and other gases could be introduced to study the flow of electrons through the tube. While experimenting with such a tube, Roentgen discovered that invisible, unknown rays were coming from the tube that caused a screen to fluoresce. This was the initial discovery of x-rays.

2. X-rays were initially used in a great variety of experiments. Images were made of animals such as frogs and lizards, to peek inside people's pockets, and to look at feet inside shoes. Only later were the possible harmful effects discovered. Present additional uses of x-rays include examining luggage at airports and checking manufactured parts for structural integrity.

3. As early as 1898 Dr. Rollins began warning people about the hazards of x-ray radiation, and radiation skin burns were fairly common among experimenters. Not until the 1940s, however, was protection from x-rays taken very seriously, leading to the development of shielding and modern approaches to protection.

4. An R/F unit is simply a combined radiographic/fluoroscopic unit, a general purpose unit that can be used for both radiography and fluoroscopy.

5. The tube can be raised and lowered, often moved back and forward on a track, and tilted at any position between horizontal and vertical. The table can be raised and lowered and usually can be tilted.

6. Chest radiographs are almost always obtained with the patient standing. Some other procedures such as exams of the acromioclavicular joint, the abdomen, and the cervical spine also have better results with the patient standing.

7. The x-ray tube housing (1) prevents the leakage of x-rays from the tube except for the primary beam through the window, (2) protects the tube when the unit is being moved and handled, and (3) supports the tube and holds it immobile during examinations. It also allows for cooling of the tube.

8. In World War I Marie Curie worked with the French government to outfit 18 cars as special mobile radiographic units for performing diagnostic examinations at the front lines.

9. Primary radiation is the useful x-ray beam itself. Protection is needed to prevent any x-rays from passing by the patient or through the patient and reaching anyone else. Secondary radiation is leakage radiation and scatter radiation. Leakage radiation consists of x-rays from the tube that are not part of the primary beam but that are not absorbed as they should be, by the tube housing. Scatter radiation is produced when x-rays from the primary beam interact with molecules inside the patient, in the air, in the film cassette or other equipment, or elsewhere and are deflected in other directions. Scatter radiation can strike anywhere in the area around the examination, and thus protection should always be used to prevent exposure for any personnel.

Answers for Applications

1. Common uses of CT scanning include imaging the brain, tumors, skeletal fractures, herniated vertebral discs, and congenital abnormalities.

2. The fundamental difference is that radiography produces static images, whereas fluoroscopy produces moving images. Radiographs are typically used to image anatomic structures, such as bones. Fluoroscopy is used when it is important to see something moving, such as a contrast medium moving through blood vessels or a catheter being introduced into some part of the body.

3. Following are some desirable characteristics of radiographic examination tables. Note that not all are present in all equipment.

   The table top can be raised and lowered (this makes it easier for patients to climb on and off while still being at a comfortable working height for the radiographer).

A floating table top moves in all directions (this makes it easier for the patient to be positioned in the best way for each specific examination).

The table top can be tilted (this is needed for some examinations).

The table top should be uniformly radiolucent (this should be true of all tables).

The table top should be easy to clean, smooth, and hard to scratch (scratches could allow material to accumulate in them, which may affect the image).

4. The three main parts are the x-ray tube, the table (usually with a Bucky tray assembly), and the control panel.

5. The most unique part of a mammography unit involves the device for positioning the breast. Breast tissue must be compressed in order to provide the best image.

6. One of the most common procedures involving the injection of contrast medium is arteriography, which shows the flow of blood through vessels to different organs, such as the brain, heart, or kidneys.

7. Mobile radiographic equipment is often used in the emergency room, the operating room, intensive care units, or the patient's hospital room to assess postsurgical condition.

8. Devices commonly used to help shield radiographers from radiation include the following:

   Lead shielding in the walls, floor, and ceiling

   X-ray tube housing

   Secondary radiation barriers (moveable or fixed), including control room windows

   Note: Many other protective devices are used but were not discussed in this module, such as personal equipment like protective aprons, thyroid shields, glasses, gloves, etc.

Radiographic Density and Contrast

Self-Assessment Pretest

Use this pretest to assess your knowledge of the material in this module before you begin to work through the following exercises. Circle the best answer for each of the following questions. The answers are at the end of this module.

1. Density is defined as which of the following?
   a. The overall amount of blackening on the film
   b. The difference in blackening between adjacent areas
   c. The amount of blackening allowed by a particular film
   d. The heaviness of a film

2. How does doubling the mAs affect the exposure rate?
   a. Cuts exposure rate in half
   b. Doubles the exposure rate
   c. Reduces the exposure rate by 15%
   d. Increases the exposure rate by 15%

3. How does increasing the kVp by 15% affect density?
   a. Cuts the density in half
   b. Doubles the density
   c. Decreases the density by 15%
   d. Increases the density by 15%

4. Increasing the SID does what to density if all other factors are unchanged?
   a. No effect on density
   b. Increases the density
   c. Decreases the density
   d. Effect depends on OID

5. An intensifying screen allows for which of the following?
   a. Reducing the patient exposure but achieving the same density
   b. Increasing the density without increasing the patient exposure
   c. Both of the above
   d. Neither of the above

6. Which part of the x-ray beam is the most intense?
   a. The part in the center
   b. The part at the circumference
   c. The part nearer the cathode
   d. The part nearer the anode

7. What is true when a grid is used?
   a. Less scatter radiation reaches the film.
   b. There is better contrast in the image.
   c. Somewhat higher exposures are required.
   d. All of the above are true.
   e. None of the above are true.

8. What does filtration improve?
   a. Less intense average quality of beam
   b. More intense average quality of beam
   c. Greater number of high-energy x-rays reach patient
   d. Lesser number of high-energy x-rays reach patient

9. What does subject contrast refer to?
   a. Variations in patient size
   b. The manufacturer of the x-ray tube
   c. The type of exam being given
   d. All of the above
   e. None of the above

10. A collimator is used to do which of the following?
    a. Attach cones to the tube housing
    b. Control the field size of the primary beam
    c. Hold the patient in position
    d. Mount the intensifying screen on the film

Key Terms

Before continuing, be sure you can define the following key terms.

Added filtration: Aluminum filters added outside the tube to increase filtration of the primary beam.

Anode heel effect: The normal variation in the intensity of the x-ray beam between the anode and cathode sides of the beam; the part of the beam nearer the anode is less intense than that nearer the cathode.

Aperture diaphragm: A nonadjustable device that restricts the size of the beam's field size as it emerges from the tube; not as commonly used as cones and collimators.

Attenuation: The reduction in the number of x-ray photons as the x-ray beam passes through matter.

Automatic processor: Film processing equipment that automatically moves the exposed film through the processing stages from developer to dryer.

Black metallic silver: The blackening in a radiographic film; exposed silver crystals in the film are converted by the processing into black metallic silver.

Characteristic curve: A measurement showing the relationship between exposure and density.

Collimator: A device, usually adjustable, that restricts the size of the x-ray beam as it emerges from the tube.

Compensating filter: A type of added filter designed to compensate for different tissue densities in different body areas by filtering the beam through one area more than through another.

Cone: A metal device shaped like a cone or cylinder that attaches below the tube port and limits the field size of the primary beam.

Contrast: The differences in density on adjacent areas of the radiograph; see **subject contrast** and **film contrast.**

Contrast medium: A substance ingested, inserted, or injected into the body to provide that body area with more contrast on the radiograph.

Densitometer: An instrument that measures film blackness.

Density: The overall amount of blackening on a radiograph; also called optical density or radiographic density.

Development fog: A generalized graying of a radiograph that results when unexposed silver crystals in the film are developed.

Fifteen percent rule: The principle that a kVp increase of 15% doubles the exposure.

Filter: A device, usually made of aluminum, inserted into the path of the x-ray beam near the tube to absorb the low-energy (long wavelength) x-rays, thereby increasing the average energy of the beam; see **inherent filtration** and **added filtration.**

Film contrast: The inherent ability of a radiographic film to record a range of densities.

Focus-film distance (FFD): The distance between the source of the x-ray beam (at the focal point) and the radiographic film; this is an older term that has generally been replaced by "source-to-image receptor distance" (SID).

Grid: A device that absorbs scatter radiation before it reaches the image receptor but allows most of the primary beam radiation to pass through.

High-energy x-rays: X-ray photons with higher energy levels, produced when the kVp is higher.

Inherent filtration: The tube elements that filter the beam, including the glass envelope and the insulating oil.

Intensifying screen: A device that converts x-ray photons to light photons to help create the latent image on the film, thereby reducing the x-ray exposure required.

mA: Abbreviation for milliamps, the measure of the flow of electrons from the cathode to the anode in an x-ray tube, which is an indirect measurement of the number of x-ray photons produced in the beam.

mAs: Abbreviation for milliamp-seconds, the product of the tube current in mA and the length of the exposure in seconds.

Pathology, pathological condition: A disease or condition; for radiographers, pathology usually refers to a condition that causes some visible change in a radiograph.

Phosphor: The crystals in an intensifying screen that emit light when struck by x-ray photons.

Scatter radiation: Radiation that results when x-ray photons in the primary beam interact with atoms inside the patient or other matter, rather than being absorbed or passing through and reaching the image receptor in a straight line; scatter radiation produces film fog.

Source-to-image receptor distance (SID): The distance between the x-ray tube and the film or other image receptor.

Subject contrast: The contrast that results from differences in tissue density in the patient.

Trough filter: A type of compensating filter to filter out more on both sides of the "trough."

Wedge filter: A type of compensating filter that gradually filters out more from one side to the other.

Topical Outline

The following material is covered in this module.

I. Density and contrast are two important characteristics of radiographs.
   A. Both density and contrast are important for diagnostic quality.
   B. Both density and contrast are affected by a number of variables within the radiographer's control.
II. Density, also called optical density or radiographic density, is the overall amount of blackening on the film. Many factors affect the density of an image.
   A. Density results when silver halide crystals in the film emulsion are exposed by x-ray photons and then converted into black metallic silver by the development process.
      1. Density varies from total black to nearly clear (unexposed).
      2. A radiograph can be overexposed (too dark) or underexposed (too light).
      3. Contrast refers to the difference between adjacent areas of darkness and lightness in the radiograph.
      4. A densitometer measures density.
   B. Exposure is a key factor determining density.
      1. The characteristic curve measures the relationship between exposure and density.
      2. mAs is the primary factor affecting density, the product of the tube current and the exposure time.
      3. The x-ray exposure rate is directly proportional to the mAs.
   C. The kVp also affects density.
      1. Increasing the kVp by 15% doubles the exposure and thus the density.
      2. Higher kVp may cause more scatter, which increases the density caused by fog.
      3. Because of other factors related to kVp — such as penetration, patient dose, scatter, and contrast — usually mAs rather than kVp is manipulated if a radiograph must be repeated because it is too light or too dark.
   D. Source-to-image receptor distance (SID) also affects density.
      1. Because of the inverse square law, the intensity of the x-ray beam decreases as the SID increases.
      2. Even slight differences in SID affect density.
   E. Intensifying screens help increase density without increasing the exposure.
      1. The phosphor layer in the intensifying screen emits light when struck by x-ray photons.
      2. The light photons produced by the screen increase the film exposure without the patient having to be exposed to as much radiation.
   F. The anode-heel effect, which causes the beam to be more intense on the cathode side than on the anode side, can be used to advantage to produce more even density when imaging certain body areas.
   G. Grids also improve density by absorbing much of the scatter radiation produced inside the patient's body.
   H. Collimators, aperture diaphragms, and cones also help reduce scatter radiation, and thereby improve diagnostic density, by restricting the size of the beam penetrating the patient.
   I. Filtration provides additional control over density.
      1. Filters absorb low-energy (long wavelength) x-rays and thereby increase the average energy of the beam.
      2. Added filtration, such as aluminum filters, adds to the inherent filtration of the tube glass port.

3. Compensating filters, such as wedge filters and trough filters, provide more filtering in one area than in another and are used to even out densities that would otherwise vary too much because of differences in body structures.

J. The patient's size and body thickness, as well as certain pathological conditions, also affect density, with larger patients and body areas requiring greater exposures to produce adequate density in the image.

K. Film processing affects density.

1. In the developing stage, density is affected by the developer time and temperature, the chemical concentration, and the size of the film crystals.

2. The fixing stage prevents the image from fading, the density from decreasing.

3. The washing and drying stages complete the process.

III. Contrast, defined as the density differences on adjacent areas of the radiograph, is important for diagnostic images.

A. Subject contrast refers to the different densities in the image resulting from attenuation differences in the body.

B. Film contrast is the inherent ability of a particular film to record a range of densities.

1. High-contrast films, also called short-scale films, show sharp differences in density — but with relatively few steps in the gray scale from light to dark.

2. Low-contrast films, called long-scale films, show more subtle differences with slight tissue variations, with more shades of gray.

C. Other factors within the radiographer's control also affect contrast.

1. Scatter radiation causes fog, which reduces the contrast in a radiograph.

a. Grids, collimators, and other beam-restricting devices reduce the amount of scatter radiation.

2. Film-screen combinations have been developed that produce the best density and contrast for different types of examinations.

3. Fog, which uniformly increases density and reduces contrast, may result from poor film storage or development conditions.

4. The use of standardized SIDs prevents density and contrast deviations that could result from inconsistent SIDs.

5. Contrast media are used to increase contrast in body areas into which the medium is injected, ingested, or otherwise inserted.

a. Positive contrast agents (such as barium ingested into the stomach) attenuate x-rays and decrease the density in that area of the radiograph.

b. Negative contrast agents (such as air injected into an organ) help to let x-rays pass through the area and increase the density in that area of the radiograph.

6. Problems with the film processing solutions can cause chemical fog that reduces contrast.

Review

1. _____, the overall amount of blackening in the radiograph, depends on the

amount of _____ that reaches a particular area of film and the amount of

_____ deposited when the film is developed.

2. Three things can happen when an x-ray photon enters a patient's body. It may be

    _____ through to reach the film, it may be _____ and not leave the

    body, or it may be _____ such that it leaves the body in a different direction.

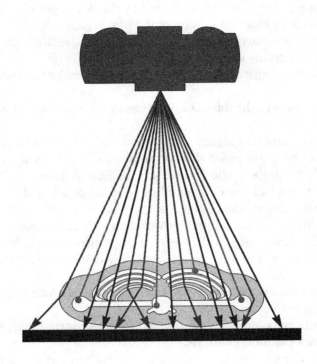

3. An instrument called a(n) _____ is used to measure density on a radiograph. The

    relationship of the _____ to density is shown by curve. For example, increasing

    the exposure would _____ the density.

4. mAs can be increased by increasing either _____ or _____ or both. The

    higher mAs _____ the density in a radiograph.

5. A setting of 100 mA and 0.2 seconds results in an mAs of _____. A setting of 200

    mA and 0.1 seconds results in an mAs of _____.

6. Increasing the kVp by 15% will _____ the density. For example, increase the kVp from 80 to _____ to double the density. Too high a kVp, however, will cause _____ radiation, which results in _____ and a lowering of contrast.

7. SID, which stands for _____, affects density also. The longer the SID, the _____ the density. Because of the inverse square law, for example, doubling the SID will reduce the density to _____ of what it was. In practice, however, the SID is usually _____ in the imaging department.

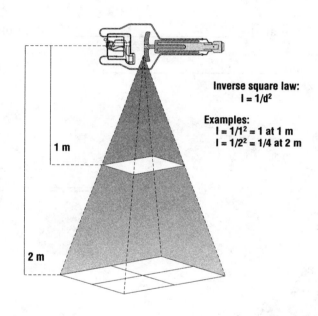

Inverse square law:
I = 1/d²

Examples:
I = 1/1² = 1 at 1 m
I = 1/2² = 1/4 at 2 m

1 m

2 m

8. When a(n) _____ screen is used, _____ x-ray photons are needed to make an exposure, because the x-ray photons interact with the _____ in the screen to produce light photons. These light photons then help expose the _____. Overall, the patient's radiation exposure is _____.

9. In some situations one can take advantage of the fact that one side of the x-ray beam is more

   intense than the other, called the _____ effect. The side of the beam nearer

   the _____ is stronger than the side of the beam nearer the _____.

   Therefore one would put the _____ side of the beam over the thicker part of

   the body.

10. A(n) _____ has shutters that can be adjusted to change the

    _____ of the primary x-ray beam. Restricting the beam helps reduce

    _____, which causes film fog.

11. Shown below to the left is a(n) _____. To the right are

    _____ and _____.

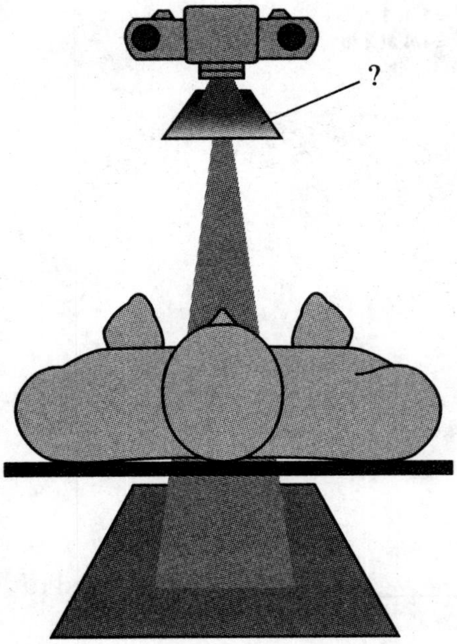

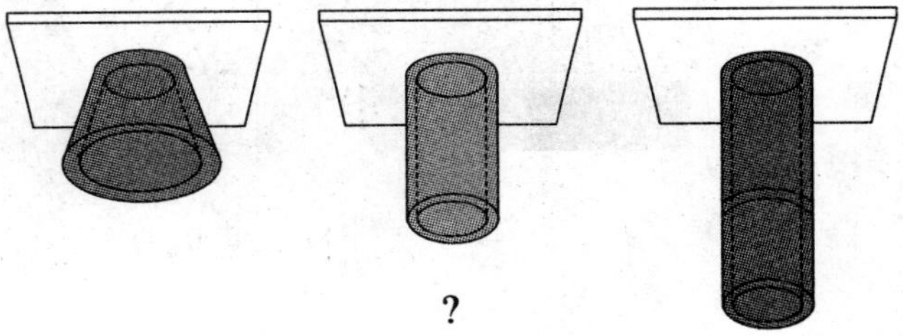

12. Added filtration _____ the low-energy, long-wavelength x-rays from the beam.

_____ filtration is part of the tube system, such as the glass port of the tube.

_____ filters are a type of added filter used to even out, or compensate for, unwanted variations in density caused by anatomical structures. The metal used in many filters is

_____, and the measurement of most added filtration is expressed in terms of

aluminum _____.

13. The developing process begins with the bath of _____ solution, in which the

exposed silver halide crystals are converted into _____. The next step,

called _____, stops the developing and makes the image permanent on the

film. Then the film is washed and _____. This whole process is handled in

_____ processors in less than 2 minutes.

STEPS INVOLVED IN PROCESSING X-RAY FILM

14. _____ contrast depends on the body size of the patient and the part being

examined, whereas _____ contrast depends on the properties of the film

being used.

15. A(n) _____ works to reduce scatter radiation by _____ scat-

tered x- ray photons, because photons cannot pass through the grid except in a(n)

_____ line from the tube.

16. Ingesting a(n) _____ medium such as barium _____ the body den-

sity in the area filled with barium, making that area on the radiograph look

_____.

Learning Quiz

The following material is similar to the interactive exercises found in the CD-ROM version of this module operated in the "Student Mode." These questions will allow you to review the concepts presented in this module and will help you to gain a more complete understanding of the material.

1. What, if anything, can be done with a radiograph that turns outs too dark or too light and is difficult to use as a diagnostic image?

2. Because of the shape of the characteristic curve, which shows the relationship of exposure and density, changes in the exposure have different effects on the density. Examine this illustration of a characteristic curve. Is the change in density greater with changes in mid-range exposure levels or at lower exposure levels?

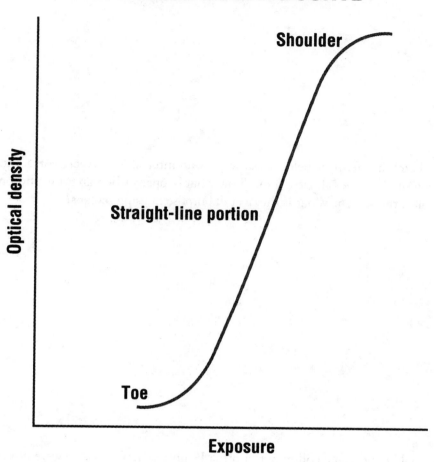

THE CHARACTERISTIC CURVE

Optical density

Shoulder

Straight-line portion

Toe

Exposure

3. Technique charts and automatic exposure control systems are both designed for the same general reason. Explain that purpose.

4. Draw a simple sketch in the space below to show how an intensifying screen works. Include a cross-section of a single screen above a film. Show what happens when an x-ray photon strikes a phosphor crystal in the screen. What is the overall purpose of using screens?

5. Explain what would happen if a collimator or other beam-restricting device were not used and the primary beam field size was larger than the film. What is the difference for the patient? What is the difference in the resultant radiograph?

6. What does "2 mm Al equivalency" refer to in a filter?

7. Why are computerized, digital images being used more commonly instead of film?

8. List the four steps that occur in an automatic film processor.

Applications

1. With all other variables staying the same, the radiographer doubles the mA setting at the control console. Describe the effects of this change in terms of the following:
   a. The current flow through the tube filament

   b. The stream of electrons from the cathode to the anode

   c. The number of x-ray photons produced

   d. The quality of the x-ray beam

   e. The density on the radiograph

2. With all other variables staying the same, the radiographer increases the kVp setting from 100 to 115. Describe the effects of this change in terms of the following:
   a. The current flow through the tube filament

   b. The potential difference (voltage) between the cathode and anode

c. The stream of electrons from the cathode to the anode

d. The number of x-ray photons produced

e. The energy levels of the x-ray photons produced

f. The density on the radiograph

3. Name the three main causes of fogging.

4. You are about to perform an examination with a mobile unit in the intensive care unit. Normally you would use an SID of 40 inches for this examination. The technique chart specifies 60 mA at this SID. Because of patient positioning difficulties and equipment around the patient that cannot be moved, however, you are forced to use a SID of 20 inches. What should the mA selection be?

5. Imagine a situation in which you are asked to use a wedge filter to even out the radiographic density for a patient's body area because an unusual pathology has greatly increased the tissue density on the patient's left side. Which part of the wedge filter should be positioned in the beam on the patient's left side?

6. Why might a positive contrast medium be used to obtain an image of the intestines?

Posttest

Circle the best answer for each of the following questions. Your instructor has the correct answers.

1. The visible blackness on a finished radiograph is composed of which of the following?
   a. Silver halide crystals
   b. Metallic silver
   c. Unexposed film emulsion
   d. Fixer

2. Contrast is defined as which of the following?
   a. The difference between adjacent areas of density in a radiograph
   b. The overall amount of blackness in a radiograph
   c. The characteristic ability of a grid to reduce scatter
   d. None of the above

3. The characteristic curve has to do with which of the following?
   a. mA and kVp
   b. mA and mAs
   c. Exposure and contrast
   d. Exposure and density

4. If a radiograph was made at 100 kVp, and you wanted to double the amount of density to make a second radiograph (with all other factors remaining unchanged), what kVp would you use?
   a. 50
   b. 85
   c. 115
   d. 200

5. What is the result of scatter radiation reaching the film?
   a. Fog
   b. More density
   c. Less contrast
   d. All of the above
   e. None of the above

6. Which factor is most often manipulated if a radiograph must be repeated because it is too light or too dark?
   a. mAs
   b. kVp
   c. SID
   d. OID

7. If all other factors remained the same, increasing the SID would have what effect on density of the radiograph?
   a. Less density
   b. More density
   c. Same density
   d. Depends on patient size

8. How is the intensifying screen usually positioned?
   a. Next to the filter
   b. Just inside the collimator
   c. On top of the patient
   d. Next to the film

9. What is the main reason for using an intensifying screen?
   a. To reduce scatter
   b. To reduce patient exposure
   c. To decrease density
   d. To make up for decreased penetration with large patients

10. Reasons to use a collimator or other beam-restricting devices include which of the following?
    a. Less scatter radiation
    b. Lower patient exposure
    c. Improved contrast
    d. All of the above
    e. None of the above

11. What do compensating filters compensate for?
    a. Differences in body structures
    b. Differences in kVp settings
    c. Variations in the cross-section of the x-ray beam
    d. Variations in SID

12. Irregularities with the film developer can cause which of the following?
    a. Poor density
    b. Poor contrast
    c. Both poor density and poor contrast
    d. Neither poor density nor poor contrast

13. Film contrast is defined as which of the following?
    a. The variations in metallic silver resulting from how much of the beam is attenuated within the patient
    b. The color range of the film
    c. The film speed multiplied by the exposure time
    d. The inherent ability of a film to record a range of densities

14. What can cause fog?
    a. Scatter radiation
    b. Improper film storage conditions
    c. Incorrect film developer temperatures
    d. All of the above
    e. None of the above

15. Which of the following is true of contrast media?
    a. They always increase the density in certain areas of the radiograph.
    b. They always decrease the density in certain areas of the radiograph.
    c. They affect the density in different ways depending on the media.
    d. None of the above are true.

Answer Key

Answers to Pretest

1. a

2. b

3. b

4. c

5. c

6. c

7. d

8. b

9. a

10. b

Answers to Review

1. Density, radiation (or x-rays or x-ray photons), black metallic silver

2. Transmitted, absorbed, scattered

3. Densitometer, exposure, increase

4. mA, exposure time (seconds), increases

5. 20 mAs, 20 mAs

6. Double, 92, scatter, fog

7. Source-to-image receptor distance, lower, one fourth, standardized

8. Intensifying, fewer, phosphor, film, lower

9. Anode heel, cathode, anode, more intense (or cathode)

10. Collimator, field size, scatter

11. Aperture diaphragm, cones, cylinders

12. Removes (or reduces), inherent, compensating, aluminum, equivalency

13. Developer, black metallic silver, fixing, dried, automatic

14. Subject, film

15. Grid, absorbing, straight

16. Contrast, increases, whiter (or lighter)

Answers to Learning Quiz

1. A film that is too dark because it was overexposed may in some cases still be useable. An optical scanner or even a very bright light may lighten the image so that the image can be seen well enough to be useful. An image that is too light from being underexposed, however, cannot be manipulated to make the image any more visible; unfortunately in this case a repeat radiograph is probably necessary.

2. As the curve shows, exposure changes at mid range levels cause bigger changes in density. Exposure changes at very low or very high levels, shown in the flatter parts of the curve in the top and bottom portions, cause smaller changes in density.

3. Technique charts and automatic exposure control systems are both designed to ensure the best contrast and density result in an examination. Technique charts accomplish this by providing the best mAs and kVp settings for different standard examinations, based on the equipment present in the radiographic suite. Automatic exposure systems work through a sensor that determines when the exposure is enough to achieve the best density and then stops the exposure.

4. You do not need to be an artist to illustrate the principle of how an intensifying screen works. The x-ray photon strikes the phosphor crystal in the intensifying screen and produces several light photons at that point, which then strike the film. Because the screen is immediately next to the film, the light photons may spread out slightly before they reach the film. The overall purpose of using screens is to reduce the patient exposure dose but still produce adequate density in the radiograph.

5. If the beam field size is larger than the film, the exposure of the patient in the area outside the film is pointless. The patient is being exposed to more radiation than necessary. The effect on the radiograph would be an overall lowering of contrast and a higher density because the extra body exposure will produce scatter radiation that may reach the film. Therefore collimators and other beam-restricting devices such as cones and cylinders are designed to reduce patient exposure.

6. "2 mm Al equivalency" states that the amount of filtering that would be achieved is the equivalent to the filtering provided by 2 mm of aluminum. Aluminum equivalency is the standard for determining the filtration effects of other materials used in filters.

7. Film is more expensive, and computerized images can also be stored more easily and efficiently on computer disk or paper. Computerized images can also be manipulated, if needed, to improve image visualization.

8. Developing, fixing, washing, drying.

Answers for Applications

1. With all other variables staying the same, doubling the mA setting causes this set of changes:
   a. The current flow through the tube filament is doubled.
   b. Twice as many electrons stream from the cathode to the anode.
   c. Twice as many x-ray photons are produced.
   d. The quality of the x-ray beam is unchanged. Remember: the quality is the energy level of the x-ray photons, which is determined by the kVp, not the mA.
   e. The density on the radiograph increases (but does not necessarily double).

2. With all other variables staying the same, increasing the kVp setting from 100 to 115 causes this set of changes:
   a. The current flow through the tube filament is unchanged—remember, that depends on mA, not kVp.
   b. The potential difference (voltage) between the cathode and anode increases from 100 to 115— that is what the kVp selection determines.
   c. The number of electrons from the cathode to the anode is unchanged (that is determined by the mA), but they are moving faster because of the greater potential difference (the attraction of the negatively charged electrons to the positively charged anode).
   d. The number of x-ray photons produced is unchanged, because this is determined by the mA, not the kVp.
   e. The energy levels of the x-ray photons produced is higher, because the kinetic energy of the faster moving electrons in the tube is higher.
   f. The density on the radiograph doubles. Remember the 15% rule: a change of 15% in the kVp doubles the density.

3. Film fogging can be caused by any of these factors:
   a. Scatter radiation reaching the film
   b. Improperly stored film (exposed to light or radiation)
   c. Poor developer conditions (developing unexposed silver crystals), including incorrect solution strength, temperature, or time

4. The mA should be 1/4 of the original mA, or 15 (1/4 of 60). Remember the inverse square law: as distance is doubled, the exposure decreases by the squared factor of four. Similarly, as the distance is cut in half, the exposure is four times as intense. Therefore the mA should be reduced to 1/4 of its original setting to compensate for this.

5. Take a moment to think this through and visualize the situation. The patient's left side has the greater tissue density. To achieve a radiographic density with both sides consistent, the thicker part of the wedge filter would be positioned in the beam on the patient's right side. That way, the less intense part of the beam goes through the "thinner" part of the body, and the more intense part of the beam goes through the "thicker" part of the body. This helps the density in the film be more balanced.

6. Positive contrast media are used when it is important to decrease the density in an area, as the x-rays through that area are more attenuated. A positive contrast medium therefore makes that area appear lighter on the radiograph. Because tissue densities of the intestines may not be different enough from other structures in the abdomen, use of a contrast agent would help make this area "stand out" on the radiograph.

Recorded Detail

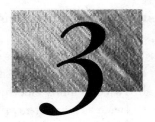

Self-Assessment Pretest

Use this pretest to assess your knowledge of the material in this module before you begin to work through the following exercises. Circle the best answer for each of the following questions. The answers are at the end of this module.

1. What is recorded detail?
    a. The degree of sharpness of structures as recorded in the radiograph
    b. The total amount of blackness on the film
    c. The difference in blackness in adjacent areas on a radiograph
    d. Penumbra

2. What is unsharpness?
    a. Another word for recorded detail
    b. The kind of fog that results from scatter when a grid is not used
    c. The blurring that occurs at the edge of structures imaged because of geometric factors
    d. The nonblurred areas in the middle of structures in the image

3. Each line pair consists of which of the following?
    a. Two lines and the space between them
    b. One line and the space next to it before the next line
    c. Two lines and two spaces
    d. One line and the space on each side of it

4. Angling the anode to the most optimal degree has what effect?
    a. Increases the production of higher energy x-ray photons and reduces scatter
    b. Reduces the focal spot size and improves recorded detail
    c. Prevents the x-ray beam from being too big
    d. None of the above

5. Magnification occurs in which of the following?
    a. With all larger focal spots
    b. With all smaller focal spots
    c. Only when the radiographer purposefully arranges for it
    d. On all radiographs

6. What does increasing the SID do?
   a. Increases the fog
   b. Decreases the fog
   c. Decreases the penumbra
   d. Increases the penumbra

7. Why is the OID almost always as short as possible?
   a. Short OID decreases magnification.
   b. Short OID decreases the penumbra.
   c. Short OID provides better recorded detail.
   d. All of the above are true.
   e. None of the above is true.

8. What is the primary reason for using an intensifying screen?
   a. Decrease patient exposure
   b. Increase recorded detail
   c. Eliminate the need for a grid
   d. Restrict the field size of the beam

9. Each x-ray photon striking the intensifying screen produces which of the following?
   a. No light photons
   b. One light photon
   c. Two light photons
   d. Many light photons

10. Which of the following is true of high speed films?
    a. They have thicker emulsion layer and bigger crystals.
    b. They require less patient exposure.
    c. They produce less recorded detail.
    d. All of the above are true.
    e. None of the above is true.

Key Terms

Before continuing, be sure you can define the following key terms.

Blur: Unsharpness in a radiograph caused by patient motion.
Focal spot: The area of the anode where x-ray photons are produced by bombardment of electrons from the cathode.
Geometric sharpness or unsharpness: Sharpness or unsharpness in an image that results from geometric factors which depend on the size of the focal spot and the SID and OID.
Intensifying screen: A device that converts x-ray photons to light photons to help create the latent image on the film, thereby reducing the x-ray exposure required.

Involuntary motion: Motion of or inside the patient that is outside the person's control, such as fluids moving through the gastrointestinal tract; compare to **voluntary motion.**

Latent image: The invisible "image" on exposed film, consisting of silver ions from the interaction with x-rays that have gravitated to sensitivity specks; the developer converts this into a manifest, or visible, image on the film by turning the silver ions into black metallic silver.

Latitude: The ability of a film to show different shades of gray, from light to black.

Line focus principle: The geometric principle by which the effective focal spot of the x-ray beam is made smaller by angling the anode, thereby achieving better recorded detail.

Line pair: A measurement unit for determining resolution, consisting of a line and a space before the next line; the number of line pairs visible per millimeter is a measure of recorded detail.

Magnification: The geometric phenomenon that the image on a radiograph is always somewhat bigger than the object or structure itself because the x-ray beam continues to disperse as it moves from the object to the image receptor.

Magnification radiography: An examination in which the object-to-image receptor distance is intentionally longer than necessary for the purpose of increasing the magnification for diagnostic purposes.

Object-to-image receptor distance (OID): The distance between the object being radiographed and the film or other image receptor.

Phosphor: The crystals in an intensifying screen that emit light when struck by x-ray photons.

Recorded detail: The degree of sharpness of structures recorded in a radiograph.

Sensitivity specks: Impurities in the film emulsion that attract silver ions produced when x-rays interact with the silver halide crystals; these clumps of silver ions are converted into black metallic silver by the development process.

Source-to-image receptor distance (SID): The distance between the x-ray tube and the film or other image receptor.

Speed: A characteristic of a film or intensifying screen, reflecting how quickly it reacts to x-rays; the speed of an intensifying screen refers to the efficiency and speed with which it absorbs x-rays and converts the energy into light photons.

Target: The area of the anode struck by electrons from the cathode; another term for the focal spot.

Target angle: The angle of the part of the anode struck by electrons from the cathode.

Unsharpness: The area of unsharpness at the edges of structures caused by geometric properties of the x-ray beam coming from the focal spot.

Visible detail The area of sharper detail in an image, away from the unsharpness at the edges of structures.

Voluntary motion: Patient motion that the person can control, such as holding still or stopping breathing momentarily by holding one's breath; compare to **involuntary motion.**

Topical Outline

The following material is covered in this module.

    I. Recorded detail is important for diagnostic-quality images.
       A. Recorded detail is the degree of sharpness of structures as recorded in the radiograph.
          1. Recorded detail is also called definition, sharpness, resolution, visible detail, or just detail.
          2. Radiographic quality depends on image sharpness, or recorded detail, along with visibility, resulting from density and contrast.
          3. Unsharpness is lack of recorded detail, or blurring, along the edges of structures; visible detail is the sharp, or unblurred, area within the edges.

B. The amount of recorded detailed is determined by the resolution, which is measured in line pairs visible per millimeter.
  1. The human eye can discern up to 5 line pairs per millimeter.
  2. Conventional screen-film combinations can resolve up to about 10 line pairs per millimeter.
II. Geometric unsharpness results from unavoidable geometric factors in how the x-ray beam is produced and interacts with the object being imaged.
  A. Geometric unsharpness occurs because the x-ray beam emerges not from a single spot in the tube but from an area.
    1. Electrons from the cathode strike the target on the anode focal spot where x-rays are produced.
    2. Because of the line focus principle, angling the anode helps decrease the effective focal spot size to improve the recorded detail. The anode is tilted at an average angle of 12 degrees.
  B. Unsharpness occurs because the edge of a structure is imaged by x-ray beams emerging from all parts of the focal point in the tube, at slightly different angles to the film, producing unsharpness.
  C. Magnification of the image occurs because the x-ray beam continues to disperse and spread out in the distance between the object and the image receptor (the OID).
    1. The magnification factor is calculated by the image size divided by the object's true size, or by dividing the source-to-image receptor distance (SID) by the source-to-object distance (SOD).
    2. Magnification radiography intentionally uses magnification when it is desirable to magnify a structure in a radiograph.
    3. Unsharpness caused by blurring is magnified as well.
  D. Increasing the SID decreases unsharpness because the x-ray beams from the focal spot do not spread out as far between the object and the film.
    1. Standardized SIDs with acceptable amounts of unsharpness are used for most routine examinations.
    2. Longer SIDs, such as the 72-inch SID used with chest radiographs, decrease unsharpness and the magnification of structures like the heart, providing better recorded detail.
  E. Decreasing the OID to the minimum distance minimizes both unsharpness and magnification. Except when magnification is intentionally desired, the patient is always positioned as close to the film as possible.
III. Intensifying screens and film also are important for recorded detail.
  A. The speed of film and intensifying screens refers to how much and how quickly they react to the x-ray photons.
  B. Slower film-screen combinations generally produce better recorded detail, but they also involve more patient exposure.
    1. Slower speeds are generally used with extremities, where exposure is not as major a concern.
    2. Faster speeds are used for larger body areas to keep patient dose minimal.
  C. Screens work by converting x-ray photons to light photons to expose the film with less radiation to the patient.
    1. Almost 100% of the exposure of the film results from the light produced in the screen, not the x-ray photons that reach the film, allowing much lower patient doses.
    2. Phosphor crystals inside the screen produce many light photons for each x-ray photon that strikes the crystal.
      a. The screen is composed of a base layer, a reflective layer (to direct all light at the film), the phosphor layer, and a protective coating.
      b. The screen is immediately next to the film, which is exposed by the light photons to create the latent image.
    3. Screens are classified by their speed, the rate at which they absorb x-rays. Screen speed is determined by the size of the phosphor crystals and the thickness of the phosphor layer. High-speed screens have larger crystals in thicker layers.

a. Fast screens reduce motion blur and reduce patient exposure. Because the crystals are larger, recorded detail is less.

b. Slower screens may be used when very fine detail is needed.

D. The characteristics of the radiographic film also affect recorded detail.

1. Faster films have thicker emulsion layers and larger silver bromide crystals.

a. Fast films require less patient exposure but produce less recorded detail.

b. Slower films require more patient exposure but produce better recorded detail.

2. Films and screens are used in standardized combinations established for different types of examinations.

IV. Blur is unsharpness in the image produced by movement of the patient during the exposure—just like in photography.

A. Voluntary motion can be minimized by asking the patient to hold still, to hold his or her breath, using restraints, etc.

B. Involuntary motion, such as movement within the gastrointestinal tract or involuntary muscle movement, cannot be prevented; the radiographer can only try to use short exposures and help the patient remain still with restraints.

C. Motion of the equipment must be prevented, so any vibration or damaged equipment should be checked to ensure the unit is working correctly and stays motionless through the examination.

Review

1. Recorded detail is the degree of _____ of structures actually recorded on the

_____ .

2. The blurring at the edges of structures on a radiograph is called _____, which results

because the _____ of the x-ray beam is an area rather than a point. The

_____ , on the other hand, is the area with less blurring in the center of structures.

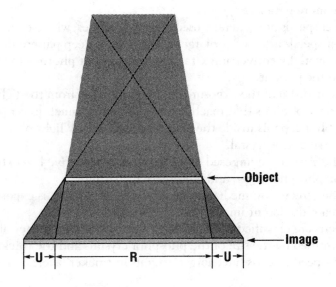

3. The amount of space on a radiograph filled by a line and the space next to it before the next line is called a(n) _____ , and this is used in the measurement of

_____ . The human eye on the average can discern about _____ line pairs per millimeter, and radiographs typically record about _____ line pairs per millimeter.

4. _____ sharpness is the term used for the mathematical relationships of the focal spot, the SID, and the OID that influence resolution. The _____ the focal spot, the greater the unsharpness. The focal spot is the area of the _____ struck by the electrons from the cathode.

IMPORTANT FACTORS FOR OBTAINING A GOOD IMAGE

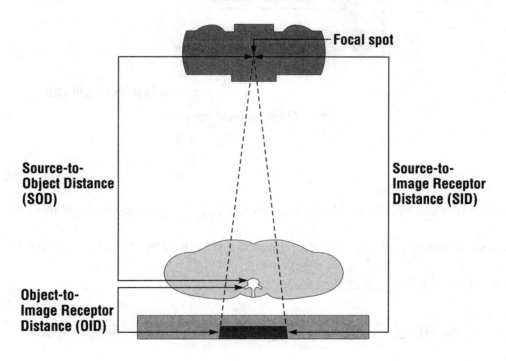

Focal spot

Source-to-Object Distance (SOD)

Source-to-Image Receptor Distance (SID)

Object-to-Image Receptor Distance (OID)

5. The _____ principle describes the relationship between the angle of the

_____ and the size of the effective _____. The average angle of the

anode is about _____ degrees.

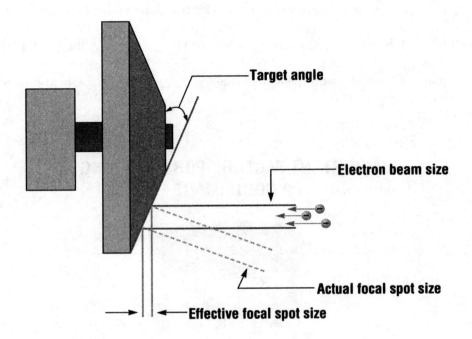

6. Magnification can be measured by dividing the _____ size by the object's actual size.

The same magnification calculation can be achieved by dividing the subject-to-image receptor

distance (SID) by the _____ .

7. Increasing the SID _____ the recorded detail because the unsharpness is

_____ . Many routine examinations are performed at an SID of _____ inches,

which has acceptable magnification and recorded detail. Chest radiographs, however, are usually

performed at an SID of _____ inches. At this larger SID, magnification _____ .

8. If the SID and focal spot size remain the same, decreasing the OID will _____ magnification. This also _____ the unsharpness and therefore _____ the recorded detail.

GEOMETRY OF MAGNIFIED IMAGE
POINT SOURCE FOCAL SPOT

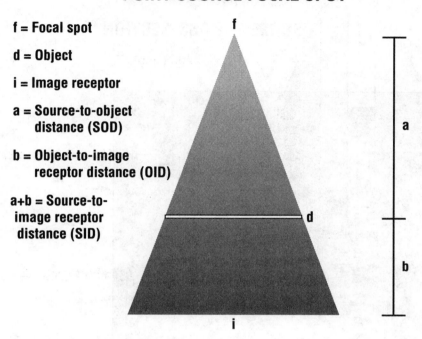

f = Focal spot

d = Object

i = Image receptor

a = Source-to-object
   distance (SOD)

b = Object-to-image
   receptor distance (OID)

a+b = Source-to-
   image receptor
   distance (SID)

9. Slow film-screen combinations are usually used for examinations of the _____, and faster film-screen combinations are used for examinations of _____ body areas.

10. Intensifying screens are used to lower the patient _____, even though they may also _____ recorded detail.

11. _____ are materials that absorb the energy of x-ray photons and emit light _____. The film is exposed primarily by the _____ .

12. The intensifying screen consists of a number of layers: a(n) _____, usually made of plastic, that supports the other layers. The next layer, the _____ layer, increases the screen's speed by reflecting light back toward the film. The _____ layer emits light photons when struck by x-ray photons. The outside _____ layer guards the screen from moisture, stains, and abrasions.

SCREEN CROSS-SECTION

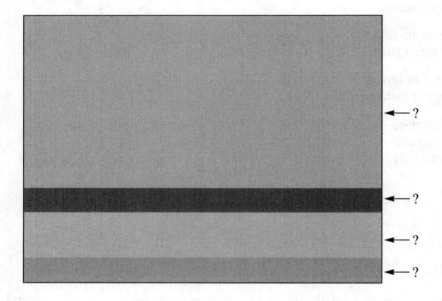

13. The resolution of an intensifying screen is determined by the size of the phosphor _____, the _____ of the phosphor layer, and the conversion efficiency for creating light photons from x-ray photons.

14. When light or x-ray photons strike a(n) _____ crystal in the film emulsion, the first step in the process of producing an image is that _____ are released that move to the sensitivity speck, giving it a negative charge. Silver ions then gravitate to the _____, and the developer turns these into _____. In this way the _____ image resulting from the radiation exposure is transformed into a manifest image.

15. The _____ of a film is its ability to show a range of different shades of gray.

16. You can help prevent a patient's _____ motion and the _____ it can cause on a radiography by giving careful instructions to the patient. The only way you can try to reduce the effects of involuntary motion, however, is to use a(n) _____ exposure.

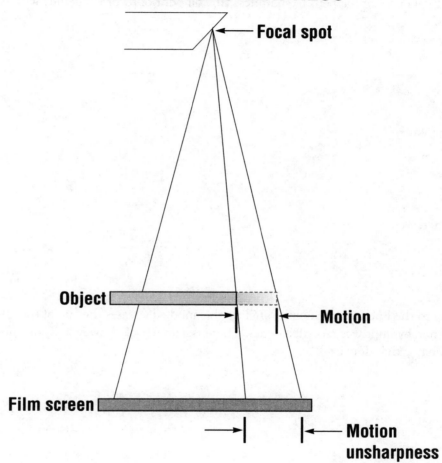

MOTION UNSHARPNESS

Learning Quiz

The following material includes interactive exercises found in the CD-ROM version of this module operated in the "Student Mode." These questions will allow you to review the concepts presented in this module and will help you gain a more complete understanding of the material.

1. What are some of the other terms that refer to recorded detail?

2. Geometric sharpness is affected primarily by three factors: the size of the focal spot, the SID, and the OID. Explain what happens to sharpness (the amount of recorded detail) with each of these changes:
   a. Focal spot increases

   b. SID increases

   c. OID increases

3. According to the line focus principle, angling the anode decreases the size of the effective focal spot and thereby improves recorded detail. There is a drawback, however, if the anode is angled too far. What is that drawback?

4. If you increase the SID and leave the OID the same, is there more or less magnification in the image? Explain the reason for your answer.

5. Why would some radiography departments switch to a 48-inch SID as the standard for most exams, rather than the traditional 40 inches? Name two benefits.

6. What is the main advantage of using an intensifying screen? What is the main disadvantage?

7. What is the effect of screen speed on recorded detail? Explain why there is a difference in recorded detail at different screen speeds.

8. Give examples of uses of very high-speed screens.

9. How is film speed the same as or different from screen speed?

10. Give three examples of involuntary patient movement.

Applications

1. Draw a cross-sectional sketch of the x-ray beam that illustrates the geometrical factors involved and the unsharpness on the film. Put a small horizontal line at the top that represents the focal spot. Put a larger horizontal line at the bottom that represents the film. Put a third, somewhat smaller line a short way above the film to represent an object. Now draw in the lines showing the edges of the beam and the resulting unsharpness. (Hint: Do not forget to draw beam lines from *both* sides of the focal spot.)

2. Magnification of the image larger than the actual object is a function of geometric factors. Working with the following variables, how big will the image on the film be?

Actual object is 10 inches across.
Distance from the tube to the film is 40 inches.
Distance from the object to the film is 2 inches.
(Hint: You need to use a calculator or long division to find the answer.)

3. You are about to perform a radiographic examination of a patient. You know that recorded detail needs to be as good a possible. Within the normal limits for the type of exam, explain how each of the following factors can affect the recorded detail and what, if anything, you can do to improve it.
   a. SID

b. OID

c. Focal spot size

d. Film-screen combination

e. Voluntary patient motion

f. Involuntary patient motion

Posttest

Circle the best answer for each of the following questions. Your instructor has the correct answers.

1. The average human eye can discern up to how many line pairs per millimeter?
   a. 1
   b. 2
   c. 5
   d. 10

2. What can be done to prevent geometric unsharpness?
   a. Increase the kVp
   b. Increase the mAs
   c. Use a higher-ratio grid
   d. None of the above

3. Why does unsharpness occur?
   a. With high kVp the central beam is too powerful and "spills over" at the edges.
   b. The edges of a structure are imaged by x-rays from both sides of the focal spot.
   c. Poor collimation does not restrict the edges of the beam.
   d. All of the above are true.

4. Why does magnification occur in all radiographs?
   a. The x-ray beam continues to spread out after passing through the patient.
   b. The focal spot is an area rather than a point.
   c. This is an unavoidable aspect of film emulsions.
   d. Light photons from the intensifying screen spread out before they reach the film.

5. How is the magnification factor calculated?
   a. The image size divided by the object's true size
   b. The SID divided by the SOD
   c. Both of the above
   d. Neither of the above

6. Why is a 72-inch SID for chest radiographs standard?
   a. A longer SID decreases penumbra.
   b. A longer SID decreases magnification of structures such as the heart.
   c. This longer SID provides better recorded detail.
   d. All of the above are true.
   e. None of the above is true.

7. If magnification was desired in a radiograph, what change would likely be made?
   a. Increase the SID
   b. Increase the OID
   c. Increase the SOD
   d. Any of the above
   e. None of the above

8. Which of the following is true of slower speed intensifying screens?
   a. They generally produce more recorded detail than faster speed screens.
   b. They generally produce less recorded detail than faster speed screens.
   c. They involve lower patient exposures.
   d. They are generally used for large body areas.

9. What percentage of the film exposure results from light photons from the intensifying screen, rather than from x-ray photons from the beam?
   a. About 1%
   b. 10%
   c. 50%
   d. Almost 100%

10. What are the advantages of high-speed screens?
    a. Lower patient exposure and reduced motion blur
    b. Lower patient exposure and more recorded detail
    c. More recorded detail and better contrast
    d. Better contrast and density

11. Which of these best describes the composition of slow-speed intensifying screens?
    a. Larger phosphor crystals, thicker layer of crystals
    b. Larger phosphor crystals, thinner layer of crystals
    c. Smaller phosphor crystals, thinner layer of crystals
    d. Smaller phosphor crystals, thicker layer of crystals

12. Which of these best describes the composition of slow-speed films?
    a. Larger silver halide crystals, thicker layer of crystals
    b. Larger silver halide crystals, thinner layer of crystals
    c. Smaller silver halide crystals, thinner layer of crystals
    d. Smaller silver halide crystals, thicker layer of crystals

13. What could help minimize blur caused by involuntary patient movement?
    a. Ask the patient to hold still
    b. Ask the patient to hold his or her breath
    c. Use short exposure times
    d. All of the above
    e. None of the above

14. Motion blur can be caused by which of the following?
    a. The patient breathing
    b. The patient's heart beating
    c. Vibration of the x-ray tube
    d. All of the above
    e. None of the above

15. Which of the following is true of film-screen combinations?
    a. They are standardized for standard examinations.
    b. They are established individually for each examination.
    c. They depend on the size of the patient.
    d. They are used only with very high kVp selections.

Answer Key

Answers to Pretest

1. a

2. c

3. b

4. b

5. d

6. c

7. d

8. a

9. d

10. d

Answers to Review

1. Sharpness (or resolution), radiograph

2. Unsharpness, focal spot, recorded (or visible) detail

3. Line pair, resolution (or sharpness, or recorded detail), 5, 10

4. Geometric, larger, anode

5. Line focus, anode, focal spot, 12

6. Image's, source-to-object distance (SOD)

7. Increases, less (or smaller), 40, 72, decreases

8. Decrease, decreases, increases

9. Extremities, larger

10. Dose (or exposure), decrease

11. Phosphors, photons, light photons

12. Base, reflective, phosphor, protective

13. Crystals, thickness

14. Silver halide, electrons, sensitivity speck, black metallic silver, latent

15. Latitude

16. Voluntary, blur, shorter

Answers to Learning Quiz

1. Other terms commonly used that refer to the amount of recorded detail are definition, sharpness, resolution, visible detail, or just detail. The term recorded detail is used because it is more precise.

2. a. With an increase in focal spot, unsharpness due to blurring increases; therefore there is less recorded detail.
   b. With an increase in SID, the unsharpness decreases, therefore increasing recorded detail.
   c. With an increase in OID, the unsharpness (and magnification) increases, therefore decreasing the recorded detail.

3. If the anode is angled too far, the beam will cover too small an area and only smaller film can be used.

4. Increasing the SID (when the OID is unchanged) will decrease the magnification because of the geometric relationships. The beam continues to spread out in every case, but the longer the SID, the less spread there is relative to the distance between the object and the image receptor (the OID). This is because of the inverse square law.

5. The longer SID both decreases magnification and increases recorded detail because there is less unsharpness.

6. The primary advantage of using an intensifying screen is that it allows using much lower exposure factors and thereby greatly decreases the patient dose. The main disadvantage is that the recorded detail may be somewhat less.

7. The faster the screen speed, the less recorded detail; the slower the screen speed, the more recorded detail. Faster screens have larger phosphor crystals in thicker layers, and therefore the resolution is not as fine because the grain is larger.

8. Very high-speed screens are used when fine detail is not a consideration and you want to limit dose. For example, high-speed screens are often used for pelvimetry, scoliosis screening, and many pediatric exams.

9. Screen speed and film speed are very similar both in how speed is determined and in how and why the speed affects recorded detail. In both cases, the speed is determined by the size of the crystals (phosphor or silver halide) and the thickness of the layer of crystals (in the phosphor layer or the film emulsion). In both cases, the larger the crystals and the thicker the layer, the faster the film or screen is—because fewer x-ray or light photons are needed to expose the crys-

tals. But because the crystals are larger, in both cases the faster speeds do not produce as fine a resolution. Slower speed films and screens have smaller crystals in thinner layers and thus are less grainy and finer in resolution, but they also both require more x-ray or light photons to expose them. Thus in both cases the slower speeds require higher patient radiation doses.

10. Examples of involuntary patient movement include the movement of fluids through the gastrointestinal tract, beating of the heart, the movement of blood through blood vessels, and breathing in an unconscious patient.

Answers for Applications

1. You don't need to be an artist to illustrate the geometrical factors that produce unsharpness. Your sketch might look something like this:

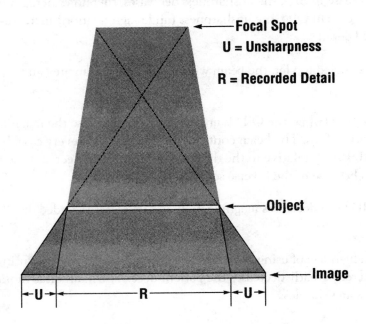

2. Here again are the variables:
   Actual object is 10 inches across.
   Distance from the tube to the film is 40 inches.
   Distance from the object to the film is 2 inches.

   Remember that the magnification factor is the SID divided by the SOD. The SID is 40. The SOD (source-to-object distance) is 40 minus 2, or 38. The magnification factor is 40 divided by 38, which equals 1.05. The image is 1.05 times bigger than the actual object, or 1.05 times 10 inches. Therefore the image on the film will be 10.5 inches across.

3. Each of the following six variables plays a role in recorded detail:

a. SID: The longer the SID, the better the recorded detail because the unsharpness is reduced. The standard settings on your department's technique charts usually produce good recorded detail, however, so you probably do not need to increase the SID beyond the standardized 40 or 72 inches for the exam.

b. OID: The smaller the OID, the better the recorded detail because the unsharpness is reduced. Therefore be sure the area of the patient being examined is as close as possible to the film or other image receptor.

c. Focal spot size: The smaller the focal spot size, the better the recorded detail. Many x-ray tubes have two different focal spot sizes. This is a variable that is usually standardized in the department for each type of examination, however, not a selection you make each time.

d. Film-screen combination: The slower the speed of the film-screen combination, the better the level of recorded detail—but the higher the patient's radiation dose. The use of different film-screen combinations is usually standardized in the department for the best results in different types of exams, not a selection you make each time, unless a variation from the standard is needed for a particular reason.

e. Voluntary patient motion: Because motion causes blur, the patient must be as still as possible. Explain to the patient why it is essential not to move during the exposure (blur could cause a need for the exam to be repeated). If the patient is uncomfortable in the position or has difficulty supporting an extremity in the right position, use pillows, sandbags, or other devices to provide support. Ask the patient to hold his or her breath at the moment of the exposure.

f. Involuntary patient motion: Because this motion too can cause blurring, your goal is to reduce its effects whenever possible, although the patient cannot voluntarily control the motion. Involuntary muscle movements may be controlled with restraints. In addition, when it is important to do so, use the shortest possible exposure to minimize the effects of any motion that does occur.

Distortion

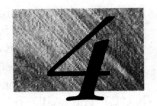

Self-Assessment Pretest

Use this pretest to assess your knowledge of the material in this module before you begin to work through the following exercises. Circle the best answer for each of the following questions. The answers are at the end of this module.

1. Distortion is caused by which of the following?
   a. Geometric factors
   b. Patient movement
   c. Scatter radiation
   d. kVp selection too high

2. What does size distortion mean?
   a. Images are smaller than the structures examined.
   b. Images are larger than the structures examined.
   c. Images are either smaller or larger than the structures examined.
   d. Images are shaped differently from the structures examined.

3. The inverse square law refers to which of the following?
   a. Shape distortion calculations
   b. Scatter radiation
   c. Amount of recorded detail
   d. The divergence of the x-ray beam

4. What does the use of a grid do?
   a. Increases magnification in the image
   b. Decreases magnification in the image
   c. Has no effect on magnification

5. How is the magnification factor calculated?
   a. SID divided by SOD
   b. SOD divided by SID
   c. SID divided by OID
   d. OID divided by SID

6. If a long bone being examined is positioned perpendicular to the central ray rather than parallel to it, the shape distortion will involve which of the following?
   a. Elongation
   b. Foreshortening
   c. Angulation
   d. Magnification

7. Shape distortion is greater with which of the following?
   a. More dense structures
   b. Less dense structures
   c. Thicker structures
   d. Thinner structures

8. When does distortion increase?
   a. When the structure is moved closer to the central ray
   b. When the structure is moved farther from the central ray
   c. When the structure is positioned directly perpendicular to the central ray
   d. All of the above

9. What should be done to minimize shape distortion?
   a. Position the body area centered on the central ray
   b. Ensure the x-ray beam is perpendicular to the image receptor
   c. Ensure the body area is parallel to the image receptor
   d. All of the above
   e. None of the above

10. The most accurate measurement of a structure's size can be ensured by which of the following?
    a. Calculating the magnification factor
    b. Using similar triangles to calculate shape and size distortion in the image
    c. Use of a radiopaque ruler
    d. All of the above
    e. None of the above

Key Terms

Before continuing, be sure you can define the following key terms.

Angulation: The situation in which the x-ray tube is not perpendicular to the body part being examined and the image receptor; angulation produces shape distortion.

Central ray: The geometric center of the x-ray beam as it exits the tube from the focal spot; the ray from which all other rays spread out as they move farther away from the tube.

Distortion: A misrepresentation of the size or shape of the part of the body being examined, as a result of geometric factors; see also **size distortion** and **shape distortion.**

Elongation: Shape distortion in which a structure appears to be longer than it actually is.

Focal spot: The area of the anode where x-ray photons are produced by bombardment of electrons from the cathode.

Foreshortening: Shape distortion in which a structure appears to be shorter than it actually is.

Inverse square law: The geometric principle that the intensity of radiation is inversely proportional to the square of the distance from the source of the radiation.

Magnification: The geometric phenomenon that the image on a radiograph is always somewhat bigger than the object or structure itself because the x-ray beam continues to disperse as it moves from the object to the image receptor; magnification is also called size distortion.

Magnification factor: The amount of magnification that occurs in an image, calculated as a ratio of the image size divided by the object's size, or the SID divided by the SOD.

Magnification radiography: An examination in which the object-to-image receptor distance is intentionally longer than necessary for the purpose of increasing the magnification for diagnostic purposes.

Object-to-image receptor distance (OID): The distance between the object being radiographed and the film or other image receptor.

Recorded detail: The degree of sharpness of structures actually recorded on the radiograph.

Shape distortion: The type of distortion in which the image of the body part is shaped differently than the actual structure, due to improper alignment of the x-ray tube, patient, and image receptor.

Size distortion: The type of distortion that results from magnification of the object in the image.

Source-to-image receptor distance (SID): The distance between the x-ray tube and the film or other image receptor.

Topical Outline

The following material is covered in this module.

I. Distortion is a misrepresentation of the size or shape of a part of the body in a radiographic image.
   A. Like recorded detail, distortion is a geometric property of the image affecting image detail.
   B. Size distortion occurs to some extent in all images because of the unavoidable magnification caused by the diverging x-ray beam.
   C. Shape distortion causes the image of the body part to be shaped differently from the object. Some degree of shape distortion is also inevitable.
II. Size distortion is magnification.
   A. Magnification occurs because the x-ray beam spreads out as it travels farther from the focal point. The image becomes larger, just as shadows are always larger than the objects making them.
   B. The x-ray beam spreads out following the inverse square law.
   C. The degree of magnification depends on the source-to-image receptor distance (SID) and the object-to-image receptor distance (OID).
      1. The greater the SID, the less the magnification.
         a. Because the SID is usually fixed (e.g., at 40 inches), increasing it can be impractical.
      2. The smaller the OID, the less the magnification.
         a. The patient is almost always positioned as close to the image receptor as possible to reduce magnification.
         b. With mammography, compression will help reduce magnification of calcifications and vessels located farther from the film.
         c. When grids are used for thick body parts to reduce scatter, the grid increases the OID and thus increases magnification.

d. Body structures farther from the image receptor are magnified more than other structures closer to the image receptor in the same radiographic image.

3. The magnification factor is a measurement of how much bigger the image size is than the object's size.

   a. Magnification factor is the ratio of the image size to the object's size.

   b. Because of the geometric principle of similar triangles, the magnification factor can be calculated as the source-to-image receptor distance (SID) divided by the source-to-object distance (SOD).

4. Magnification radiography is the intentional use of magnification to enlarge smaller structures in an image.

   a. A small focal spot is used to reduce the amount of blur that could affect the magnified structure.

   b. Grids are not used with magnification radiography because the air gap diverts much of the scatter radiation before it reaches the image receptor.

III. Shape distortion arises from several factors and takes different forms.

A. Shape distortion occurs as either elongation or foreshortening of a structure.

   1. Elongation is shape distortion in which the object appears longer than it really is.

   2. Foreshortening is shape distortion in which the object appears shorter than it really is.

B. Evaluating shape distortion is more subjective and depends on understanding human anatomy and the normal appearances of body parts.

C. Because of geometric factors, shape distortion results from a number of factors.

   1. Thicker objects or structures cause more distortion because the greater distance from the top to the bottom in relation to the distance to the image receptor results in the diverging x-ray beam striking these aspects of the structure at different angles.

   2. Distortion results if the central ray is not perpendicular to the image receptor.

   3. Distortion results if the body part is not positioned parallel to the image receptor.

   4. Distortion results if the central ray is not centered on the anatomy being imaged, because off-centering causes uneven divergence of the x-ray beam through the different parts of the structure; the farther a part is from the central ray, the greater the distortion.

      a. The divergence of the x-ray beam can be used to advantage in some exams such as lumbar spine exams visualizing intervertebral disk spaces.

   5. Distortion results if the image receptor is not perpendicular to the central ray and parallel to the part being examined, or is off-center.

   6. Angling the x-ray beam causes distortion but may be done intentionally for better imaging of a certain structure.

D. Special techniques can minimize shape distortion or its effects.

   1. Radiopaque rulers positioned alongside a structure can provide a true measurement even when shape (and size) distortion occur.

   2. Using several spot exposures along an extremity, each with the central ray perpendicular to the structure, can involve less distortion than one larger image with more distortion.

Review

1. A misrepresentation in an image of an object's size or shape is called _____. The less the distortion, the better the recorded _____. As magnification increases, recorded detail _____.

2. The two types of distortion are _____ distortion and _____ distortion. Size distortion is also called _____.

3. Shape distortion is called _____ when a structure appears longer in an image than the structure really is, and _____ when the structure appears shorter.

4. Magnification can be kept minimal with a(n) _____ SID and a(n) _____ OID. The _____ law describes how the x-ray beam diverges, the principle that accounts for magnification.

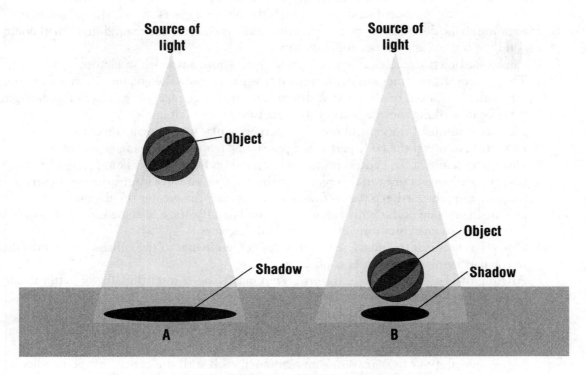

The shadow in A is larger because the object is closer to the light.

5. Mammography equipment compresses breast tissue to minimize _____ .

6. OID is kept as _____ as possible to reduce magnification. Use of a grid _____ the OID and thus increases the _____ of the image.

7. To calculate the magnification factor, divide the _____ distance by the

_____ distance. This ration equals the size of the image divided by the size of

the _____.

8. Thicker structures cause more shape distortion because the distance from the top edges of the

object to the _____ is greater than from the _____ edges. The x-ray beam con-

tinues to _____ between the top and bottom edges before it strikes the

_____, causing greater distortion.

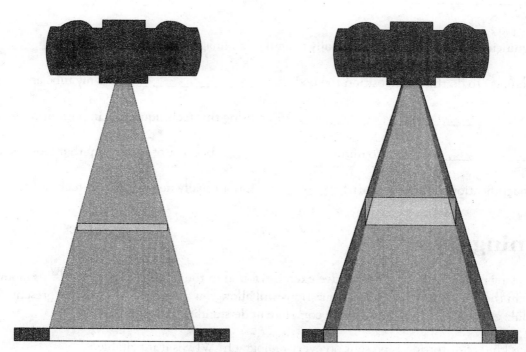

**Thick objects are unevenly magnified and their
images are more distorted.**

9. To minimize shape distortion, center the part being examined under the _____, mak-

ing sure the part is _____ to the image receptor. Avoid any _____ of the x-

ray tube. Distortion increases with body structures _____ from the central ray.

10. Determining accurate size measurements from images is difficult, particularly with the _____ bones, because the ends of the bones are farther away from the _____. Using a(n) _____ is one way to obtain accurate measurements. Another way to minimize shape distortion is to use a series of _____ exposures along a structure rather than one larger exposure.

11. Incorrect positioning of the image receptor includes not having it _____ to the part being examined, or parallel but off-_____. The tube must also be positioned to avoid _____.

12. Magnification radiography intentionally magnifies an image to improve the view of _____ structures. To do this, you position the body part _____ the x-ray tube and farther from the _____. When using this technique, it is important to use a(n) _____ focal spot to minimize _____. Because of the air gap that reduces scatter in magnification radiography, a(n) _____ is not usually needed for this technique.

Learning Quiz

The following material includes interactive exercises found in the CD-ROM version of this module operated in the "Student Mode." These questions will allow you to review the concepts presented in this module and will help you gain a more complete understanding of the material.

1. What kind of distortion is present on every radiograph? Why is it inevitable?

2. List at least four of the causes of shape distortion.

3. Describe the effects of changes in SID and OID on the amount of magnification in an image.

4. Why is it more difficult to have a very short OID when imaging thick body parts?

5. On a postero-anterior (PA) chest radiograph, which ribs will be magnified more, the anterior ribs or the posterior ribs? Why?

6. What two things can go wrong if the anatomy to be imaged is positioned off-center from the central ray?

7. What could happen if a large focal spot were used when imaging a tiny structure using magnification technique?

Applications

1. Explain the difference between two sets of factors that influence the diagnostic quality of radiographs:

Photographic qualities: contrast and density
Geometric qualities: recorded detail and distortion

2. If SID is increased, this will decrease magnification, but what is the effect on the amount of radiation the patient experiences? What is done with exposure factors to counteract this effect?

3. If a bone measures 11 cm long on the image but is actually only 10 cm long, what is the magnification factor?

4. In the following examination it is important to calculate the true size of a structure inside the body. On the image, the structure measures 2.2 inches in diameter. The SID for the examination was 40 inches. You estimate the distance from that structure within the body to the image receptor was 5 inches. What is your calculation for the true size of the structure in the body?

5. If a metal ruler 12 inches long is radiographed, positioned such that the central ray is at the 3-inch mark, what part of the ruler will look *widest* in the image? Explain why.

6. If you needed images of both the knee and ankle joint, why would you have less distortion using two spot films rather than one larger image of that whole part of the leg?

7. Imagine again a metal ruler 12 inches long being radiographed. The central ray is positioned over the halfway point at the 6-inch mark. One end of the ruler is lifted 5 or 6 inches off the image receptor (in the direction of the tube). What distortion will occur in the image? Will the image of the ruler be longer or shorter than its actual 12-inch length?

8. One more time, imagine this 12-inch ruler being radiographed. The central ray is positioned over the halfway mark at the 6-inch mark. The tube is perpendicular to the ruler. This time, one edge of the film is dropped down, angled farther away from the ruler and the tube. What kind of distortion will occur now? (Hint: Make a sketch of the spreading x-ray beam and the ruler and film, and you should be able to easily determine what will happen.)

9. Finally, place the 12-inch ruler on top of the image receptor so that it is parallel. This time, angle the x-ray tube so that the beam reaches the ruler and image receptor from above and to one side. Position the central beam at the 6-inch mark. Now what kind of distortion will occur in the image? (Again, sketching this out will help you visualize the factors involved.)

Posttest

Circle the best answer for each of the following questions. Your instructor has the correct answers.

1. Which statement is true about distortion?
   a. Distortion can be eliminated by careful positioning.
   b. Distortion can be reduced by careful positioning.
   c. Distortion can be eliminated by controlling exposure factors.
   d. Distortion can be reduced by controlling exposure factors.

2. What is the effect of scatter radiation on distortion?
   a. Scatter increases distortion.
   b. Scatter decreases distortion.
   c. Scatter and distortion are unrelated.
   d. The effect of scatter on distortion depends on other factors.

3. Which statement is true?
   a. Magnification always occurs.
   b. Magnification occurs only with elongation.
   c. Magnification occurs only when you increase the OID to image small structures.
   d. Magnification occurs only with an SID shorter than the standard SIDs used.

4. The SID divided by the SOD equals which of the following?
   a. The SOD plus the OID
   b. The OID divided by the SOD
   c. The image size divided by the object size
   d. The object size divided by the image size

5. How can the formula for calculating the magnification factor be used?
   a. To calculate object size when image size, SID, and SOD are known
   b. To calculate image size when object size, SID, and OID are known
   c. To calculate SOD when image size, object size, and SID are known
   d. All of the above
   e. None of the above

6. Which statement is true about using a grid?
   a. Size distortion increases.
   b. Size distortion decreases.
   c. Shape distortion increases.
   d. Shape distortion decreases.

7. Positioning an extremity parallel to the image receptor and perpendicular to the x-ray beam helps minimize what?
   a. Elongation
   b. Foreshortening
   c. Angulation
   d. All of the above
   e. None of the above

8. In an exam of the arm from elbow to fingertips, positioning the central ray over the wrist causes the greatest image distortion at which of the following?
   a. The fingertips
   b. The wrist
   c. The elbow
   d. The distortion is the same for all.

9. With all other factors being equal, which structure will be most distorted on an image?
   a. Dense bone
   b. Less dense muscle tissue
   c. Air-filled lungs
   d. All distorted equally
   e. None distorted

10. A radiopaque ruler can be used to do which of the following?
    a. Measure the amount of recorded detail
    b. Measure density of adjacent image areas
    c. Measure OID when positioning the patient
    d. Determine the true size of a structure in an image

11. Which statement is true?
    a. Angulation of the x-ray tube should be avoided except for a special purpose.
    b. Angulation of the x-ray tube has no effect as long as the body part and image receptor are parallel.
    c. Angulation of the x-ray tube has no effect as long as the central ray is perpendicular to the body part.
    d. All of the above are true.
    e. None of the above is true.

12. When imaging some internal structures (for example, the intestines) that cannot be positioned in a parallel plane perpendicular to the central ray, distortion can best be evaluated in terms of which of the following?
    a. An understanding of anatomy
    b. Using similar triangles to calculate distances and thus distortion
    c. The formulas for calculating the magnification factor
    d. None of the above

13. Why might off-centering the central ray from the anatomy being examined be done intentionally?
    a. To magnify small vessels
    b. To increase contrast when a grid is being used
    c. To compensate for tissue density differences
    d. All of the above
    e. None of the above

14. A radiograph taken with a child lying on his back shows the images of two pennies the child has swallowed. What is known about the penny that looks smaller?
    a. It has been in the stomach longer.
    b. It is closer to the image receptor.
    c. It is farther from the image receptor.
    d. None of the above is true.

15. Assuming the central ray is perpendicular to the image receptor and passes through the center of a long bone, in which of these situations will the long bone's image be the longest?
   a. With the long bone parallel to the image receptor
   b. With the long bone perpendicular to the image receptor
   c. With the long bone angled midway between the image receptor and the central beam
   d. All are the same

Answer Key

Answers to Pretest

1. a

2. c

3. d

4. a

5. a

6. b

7. c

8. b

9. d

10. c

Answers to Review

1. Distortion, detail, decreases

2. Size, shape, magnification

3. Elongation, foreshortening

4. Long, short, inverse square

5. Magnification

6. Short, increases, magnification

7. Source-to-image receptor, source-to-object, object (or structure)

8. Image receptor (or film), bottom, diverge (or spread out), image receptor (or film)

9. Central ray, parallel, angulation, farther away

10. Long, central ray, radiopaque ruler, spot

11. Parallel, center, angulation

12. Small, closer to, image receptor (or film), small, blur, grid

Answers to Learning Quiz

1. Size distortion, or magnification, is inevitable in all radiographs because there is always some distance between the object and the image receptor. In this distance the x-ray beams continue to diverge, spreading out, making the image larger than the object.

2. Shape distortion results from a number of causes:
   • Thicker objects or structures cause distortion because of the distance from the top to the bottom in relation to the distance to the image receptor.
   • Distortion results if the central ray is not perpendicular to the image receptor.
   • Distortion results if the body part is not positioned parallel to the image receptor.
   • Distortion results if the central ray is not centered on the anatomy being imaged, because off-centering causes uneven divergence of the x-ray beam through the different parts of the structure.
   • Distortion results if the image receptor is not perpendicular to the central ray and parallel to the part being examined, or is off-center.

3. The longer the SID, the less the magnification. The shorter the OID, the less the magnification.

4. Thick body parts often require using a grid to reduce scatter, and the grid between the patient and the image receptor increases the OID. Therefore there is more magnification in the image.

5. The posterior ribs will be magnified more because these are closer to the tube and farther from the image receptor. The x-ray beam spreads out more from these ribs to the image receptor, making greater magnification.

6. If the anatomy to be imaged is positioned off-center from the central ray, distortion will be greater. Also, some of the essential anatomy may not be included in the image, requiring that another exposure be performed.

7. Because a larger focal spot causes more blur, the blur of a small structure could obliterate the image of that structure.

Answers for Applications

1. Photographic qualities are related to factors having to do with film and exposures(radiographs are in this sense like photographs. Contrast and density both involve the type of film, the intensity of the exposure, the use of intensifying screens, grids, and filters(all variables affecting the photographic quality of the image.

Geometric properties, on the other hand, involve geometric factors such as the size of the focal spot, the inevitable blur caused by penumbra, and the inevitable magnification caused by the divergent x-ray beam. These geometric factors also include shape distortion resulting from the geometry of structures imaged within the central beam and away from it where x-rays are directed at a different angle.

Both sets of factors influence the quality of the image, but the effects of geometric variables cannot be completely eliminated because they are inherent in the radiographic imaging process.

2. If SID is increased, the amount of radiation the patient experiences is diminished because of the inverse square law: the intensity of the x-ray beam is inversely related to the distance from the tube. Because the intensity is lower, exposure factors must be increased in order to obtain enough density in the image.

3. If a bone measures 11 cm long on the image but is actually only 10 cm long, the magnification factor is calculated as the image size divided by the object size, or 11 divided by 10, or 1.1 (110%).

4. Here again are the variables:

   On the image, the structure measures 2.2 inches in diameter.
   The SID for that structure was 40 inches.
   The estimated distance from the structure to the image receptor was 5 inches.

   First calculate the magnification factor, using the formula SID divided by SOD. That is, 40 divided by 35. The magnification factor is 1.14 (114%).

   Remember that the magnification factor also equals the image size divided by the object's size. Therefore 2.2 divided by X (object size) equals 1.14.

   Mathematically, multiply both sides of the equation by 1.14, and you have X = 2.2 divided by 1.14, producing an answer of 1.93.

   The true size of the structure is 1.93 inches in diameter.

   The formula expressing all these relationships is:

   $$\frac{\text{Image size}}{\text{Object size}} = \frac{\text{SID}}{\text{SOD}}$$

5. If a metal ruler 12 inches long is radiographed, positioned such that the central ray is at the 3-inch mark, the end of the ruler at the 12-inch mark will look *widest* in the image. This is because that end of the ruler is farther away from the central ray than the other end, and the farther away an object or structure is, the greater the magnification because the x-ray beam is diverging more at that point.

6. Remember that distortion increases farther away from the central ray. With one large image of the leg, both joints will be some distance from the central ray and therefore will be distorted. But if two spot films were done instead, the central ray could be positioned over the joint in both cases, minimizing distortion.

7. In this case the image of the ruler will be shorter than its true length, as foreshortening will occur. Remember the experiment of holding the pencil at different angles—how it will look shorter when one end is farther away? Note that in this case the end of the ruler that is closer to the tube will also be magnified more than the other end, because the SID is less and the OID is more. Therefore, in addition to the foreshortening, the higher end of the ruler will be wider in the image.

8. In this case the image of the ruler will be longer than its true length, because the edge of the film that has been lowered is now farther from the object, allowing the x-ray beam to continue to diverge farther outward. That end of the ruler will also be wider than the other end, because the greater OID on that end results in greater magnification.

9. This situation at first may seem similar to the preceding one, although it is not exactly the same. Because of the angulation of the tube, even with the central ray at the 6-inch mark, one end of the ruler will be much closer to the tube than the other. Yet the ruler is flat on the film, so that the OID is the same at both ends of the ruler. The end that is farther away, therefore, will be magnified less in the image because its SID is longer, and the end closer to the tube, with a shorter SID, will be magnified more and look wider than the other end.

Beam Limitation and Filtration

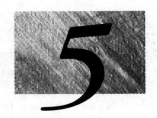

Self-Assessment Pretest

Use this pretest to assess your knowledge of the material in this module before you begin to work through the following exercises. Circle the best answer for each of the following questions. The answers are at the end of this module.

1. What can happen to an x-ray photon when it reaches the patient?
   a. It can pass directly through the patient.
   b. It can be absorbed by the body.
   c. It can scatter in another direction.
   d. All of the above are true.
   e. None of the above is true.

2. Which of the following is true?
   a. The larger the field size, the less scatter is produced.
   b. The larger the field size, the more scatter is produced.
   c. The larger the field size, the higher the contrast on the film.
   d. The larger the field size, the lower the density on the film.

3. Increasing kVp has what effect?
   a. Increases the field size
   b. Decreases the field size
   c. Decreases the amount of scatter
   d. Increases the amount of scatter

4. What is the goal of beam limitation technique?
   a. To obtain a good diagnostic image
   b. To reduce the patient exposure
   c. To reduce the amount of fog
   d. All of the above
   e. None of the above

5. A cone is a type of which of the following?
   a. Aperture diaphragm
   b. Collimator
   c. Filter
   d. Image receptor

6. Advantage(s) of collimators over aperture diaphragms include which of the following?
   a. They reduce scatter radiation more.
   b. They have a light to aid in positioning the patient.
   c. They are easier and quicker to use.
   d. All of the above are true.
   e. None of the above is true.

7. The pairs of shutters in collimators can be controlled independently to create which of the following?
   a. Different levels of radiation intensity
   b. Different filtration levels
   c. Different field sizes
   d. Different SIDs

8. The light inside the collimator is used to do which of the following?
   a. Help expose the film
   b. Activate the intensifying screen
   c. Help position the patient properly
   d. All of the above
   e. None of the above

9. Filters are used to remove which x-ray photons from the beam?
   a. Low-energy photons
   b. High-energy photons
   c. Both high- and low-energy photons
   d. Either high- or low-energy photons, depending on the type of filter

10. The main purpose of compensating filters is to do which of the following?
    a. Reduce patient exposure
    b. Harden the x-ray beam
    c. Narrow the field
    d. Provide more uniform density in the image

Key Terms

Before continuing, be sure you can define the following key terms.

Added filtration: Filters, usually made of aluminum, added outside the tube to increase filtration of the primary beam.

Aluminum equivalency: A measurement of the filtering capacity of a filter by comparing it to the filtration provided by aluminum.

Aperture diaphragm: A nonadjustable device that restricts the size of the beam's field size as it emerges from the tube; not as commonly used as cones and collimators.

Beam limitation technique: The use of any beam-limiting device to restrict the beam's size to that appropriate for the examination and thereby to reduce scatter and unnecessary patient exposure.

Central ray: The geometric center of the x-ray beam as it exits the tube from the focal spot.

Collimator: A variable-aperture beam-limiting device that uses shutters to reduce the field size, also incorporating a light and mirror to project a light beam where the x-ray beam will be, to assist in patient positioning.

Compensating filter: A type of added filter designed to compensate for different tissue densities in different body areas by filtering the beam through one area more than through another.

Compton scatter, Compton effect: A type of interaction between an x-ray photon and an atom in the patient or other matter, in which the x-ray photon passes through the matter but is deflected in a different direction; also called scatter radiation.

Cone: A type of aperture diaphragm, shaped like a cone, that attaches below the tube port and limits the field size of the primary beam.

Cone cutting: Obstruction of the x-ray beam by the edge of a cone, resulting from poor positioning of the equipment.

Contrast: The differences in density on adjacent areas of the radiograph; see **subject contrast** and **film contrast.**

Cross hairs: The device within a collimator, as part of the light localizer system, that shows the exact center of the x-ray beam.

Cylinder: A type of aperture diaphragm, shaped like a cylinder, that attaches below the tube port and limits the field size of the primary beam.

Density: The overall amount of blackening on a radiograph; also called optical density or radiographic density.

Field size: The primary x-ray beam after it has been restricted by a collimator or other device.

Filtration: The use of devices to remove some of the x-ray photons from the x-ray beam; consists of inherent filtration, added filtration, and compensating filters.

Focal spot: The area of the anode where x-ray photons are produced by bombardment of electrons from the cathode.

Fog: A generalized darkening of the image such as is caused by scatter radiation.

Half-value layer: A measurement of filtration; one half-value layer is the thickness of aluminum required to cut the intensity of the x-ray beam in half.

Hardening: Refers to the use of filtration to remove low-energy x-rays from the beam and thereby raise the average energy level.

Inherent filtration: The tube elements that filter the beam, including the glass envelope and the insulating oil.

Lead blocker: A lead sheet positioned to absorb some of the scatter radiation produced in a patient's body.

Light localizer: The part of the collimator, consisting of the light source, mirror, and cross hairs, that projects a light beam to indicate the field size and aid in positioning a patient.

Off-focus radiation: Radiation that originates in the x-ray tube at a site other than at the focal spot, which can produce image shadows.

Positive beam limitation device (PBL): A device required in fixed radiographic equipment manufactured after 1974 that automatically reduces the size of the x-ray beam to be appropriate for the image receptor.

Scatter radiation: Radiation that results when x-ray photons in the primary beam interact with atoms inside the patient or other matter and are deflected in all directions; scatter radiation produces film fog.

Shutters: The movable parts inside a collimator that allow for changing the field size.

Stem radiation: See off-focus radiation.

Total filtration: The total of added and inherent filtration.

Trough filter: A type of compensating filter to filter out more radiation on both sides of the "trough."

Unsharpness: The area of unsharpness at the edges of structures caused by geometric properties of the x-ray beam coming from the focal spot.

Wedge filter: A type of compensating filter that gradually filters out more radiation from one side to the other.

Topical Outline

The following material is covered in this module.

I. The x-ray beam is limited and filtered to get the best possible images.
   A. Scatter radiation produced in the body adds fog to the image.
      1. Scatter radiation occurs as a result of Compton interactions of x-ray photons and atoms in the body.
      2. Scatter radiation that reaches the image receptor causes a generalized increase in density, which also diminishes contrast in the image.
   B. Scatter can be reduced by various techniques.
      1. Because thinner body areas produce less scatter, compressing tissue when practical causes less scatter to be produced.
      2. Decreasing kVp tends to reduce scatter, but if kVp is too low, the low-energy photons will be absorbed in the body, increasing patient dose, without contributing to the image.
      3. The smaller the field size, the less scatter radiation is produced inside the patient, and consequently the less fog there is in the image. Therefore beam-restricting devices are used to control the field size.

II. Early beam-restricting devices included aperture diaphragms, cones, and cylinders.
   A. A fixed aperture diaphragm is a flat lead plate with a hole in it through which the x-ray beam passes; the aperture diaphragm is attached to the x-ray tube housing.
      1. Aperture diaphragms can be of any size or shape.
      2. Aperture diaphragms are easy to use but have several disadvantages.
         a. Because they are mounted close to the tube, they produce more unsharpness in the image.
         b. They allow some off-focus radiation to reach the film, producing image shadows.
         c. Unlike collimators, aperture diaphragms do not have a light guide to aid in positioning the patient.
   B. Cones and cylinders are types of aperture diaphragms shaped for specific applications.
      1. Cones and cylinders are used in dental radiography and for certain specific types of

examinations.

    2. A problem called cone cutting can occur if the equipment is not properly aligned and the cylinder or cone blocks a part of the x-ray beam needed for the image.

III. Collimators are the most commonly used beam-limiting devices today.

    A. Also called variable-aperture collimators, these devices have advantages over aperture diaphragms.

        1. Collimators do a better job of controlling field size to protect the patient from unnecessary radiation and to control scatter radiation.

        2. They include a light system to aid in patient positioning.

        3. They are quick and easy to use.

    B. Two pairs of shutters control the field size.

        1. The entrance shutters closest to the tube control for off-focus radiation that can cause image shadows.

        2. The second-stage shutters are farther from the tube and therefore reduce the unsharpness while restricting the field size.

        3. The shutters are easily controlled to a precise field size.

        4. Collimator settings are typically predetermined for standard examinations.

    C. The light localizer system within a collimator aids in patient positioning.

        1. A light within the collimator reflects from a mirror to project a light beam in the same area as the x-ray beam.

        2. Cross hairs show the exact position of the central ray.

    D. A positive beam limitation device (PBL) has been required in all fixed radiographic equipment since 1974.

        1. The PBL automatically adjusts the collimator shutters to ensure that the field size is appropriate for the size of the film cassette.

        2. Even with the PBL, the radiologic technologist must ensure the appropriate field size is chosen for the particular examination.

IV. Filtration removes some of the x-ray photons from the beam.

    A. Filtration is desirable to eliminate some of the low-energy x-ray photons that do not contribute to the image but are most likely absorbed by the body, increasing the patient dose. This is called hardening the beam.

    B. Inherent filtration is inherent in the radiographic equipment: the filtration provided by the glass tube and the insulating oil.

    C. Added filtration, usually in the form of aluminum sheets, can be added to further filter the beam.

        1. Filtering capacity is typically measured in aluminum equivalency or half-value layer — the thickness of the aluminum to reduce the intensity of the beam by half.

        2. The National Council on Radiation Protection (NCRP) sets standards for minimum levels of total filtration.

    D. Compensating filters are used in some situations to produce better diagnostic images by evening out the density when there are great variations in tissue densities.

        1. Wedge filters filter more at one end than the other, as might be used with a foot exam.

        2. Trough filters filter more at the edges and less down the middle, as might be used in a spine exam.

        3. Other specialized filters include bowtie and conic filters, as well as lead- impregnated Plexiglas filters.

Review

1. Because of the Compton effect, _____ radiation occurs from interactions within the

   body and produces generalized darkening of the film, called _____. _____ the field

   size can help decrease fog. This is one reason beam-_____ devices are used.

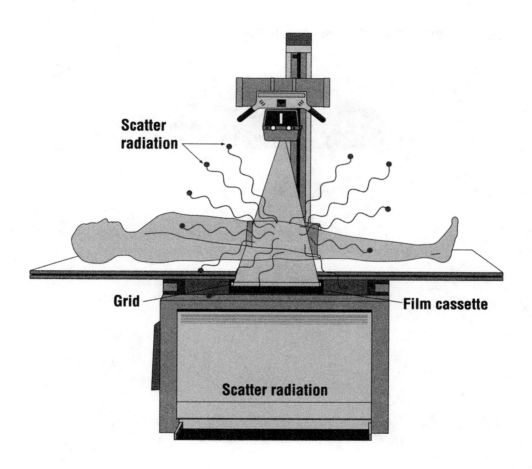

2. The thicker the patient or body area, the _____ scatter radiation is likely.

   _____ of the tissue or body part therefore helps reduce the fog resulting from scatter.

3. The _____ the kVp, the more scatter is likely to reach the _____. Yet using a low kVp is not always a solution because the patient dose is _____ if the mAs is _____ to compensate for the lower kVp.

4. Aperture _____ are usually made of _____ and are attached to the _____. The opening allows the beam to form a field size slightly _____ than the size of the image receptor.

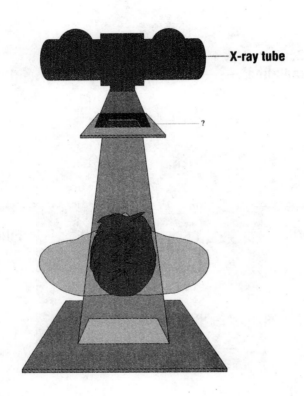

5. Because aperture diaphragms are positioned close to the tube, _____ is produced around the edges of the image. Some _____ radiation, also called stem radiation, may also reach the film. These limitations are less problematic when a _____ is used instead of an aperture diaphragm.

6. The three main parts of a collimator are pairs of _____, a(n) _____, and a(n) _____ . The shutters are usually made of _____. The first set of shutters, called the _____ shutters, help control off-focus radiation. The second set of shutters are located farther from the tube to help reduce _____.

7. The light _____ part of the collimator offers another advantage, making it easier to position the tube, the _____, and the patient. The _____ show the exact center of the beam.

8. The automatic system using a(n) _____, built into fixed radiographic equipment since 1974, determines the field size automatically based on the size and placement of the _____.

9. Filtration results in _____ of the x-ray beam because _____-energy photons are filtered out, thereby _____ the overall intensity of the beam. These low-energy photons do not contribute to the _____ but only increase the _____ because they are likely to be absorbed.

10. Inherent filtration along with _____ filtration equals total filtration. The filtering capability of a filter made of any substance, based on a comparison with aluminum, is called _____. Another measure of filtration is the _____ layer, which refers to the thickness of aluminum required to cut the intensity of the beam in half.

11. _____ filters are so named because they make up for the uneven rate at which different body parts absorb radiation. Wedge and _____ filters are two common types of compensating filters. Transparent filters made of lead-impregnated _____ are another common type, allowing the light from the collimator to pass through the filter to help position the patient.

Learning Quiz

The following material includes interactive exercises found in the CD-ROM version of this module operated in the "Student Mode." These questions will allow you to review the concepts presented in this module and will help you gain a more complete understanding of the material.

1. Describe what happens when an x-ray photon enters an atom and experiences the Compton effect.

2. Give an example of how tissue can be compressed to reduce the amount of scatter radiation occurring from that tissue.

3. List at least three disadvantages of aperture diaphragms compared to collimators.

4. Explain why two pairs of shutters are used in most collimators, and name them. What different functions do these pairs perform?

5. Make a simple sketch of a collimator showing where the light source and mirror are positioned so that the light localizing beam matches the position of the x-ray beam.

6. Why is filtering the x-ray beam often called "hardening" the beam? In what sense is the beam "harder?"

7. From everything you understand about filtering, speculate why aluminum is a popular material for making filters. This question is only partially covered in this module — but use your imagination and see if you can extrapolate at least three advantages of aluminum as a material.

8. Why would the National Council of Radiation Protection (NCRP) recommend minimum levels of filtration?

9. Describe a pathological condition of the chest that might be a basis for using a compensating filter in a chest examination to even out the density of the image.

Applications

1. Lower kVp selections generally produce less scatter radiation. So why not always use a low kVp? Explain why not and describe the radiologic technologist's goal for selecting the kVp.

2. Give examples of at least two uses of cones and cylinders as beam-restricting devices.

3. Explain how a positive beam limitation device (PBL) works automatically to ensure the field size does not exceed the film size.

4. Describe an example of when a wedge filter might be used and explain why.

5. What is a key advantage of a compensating filter made of lead-impregnated Plexiglas?

Posttest

Circle the best answer for each of the following questions. Your instructor has the correct answers.

1. What is the main problem with scatter radiation?
   a. Long exposures required
   b. Increased patient radiation dose
   c. Fog on the image
   d. All of the above
   e. None of the above

2. What affects how much scatter is produced?
   a. The size and thickness of the body area examined
   b. The tissue density of the body area examined
   c. The kVp selection
   d. All of the above
   e. None of the above

3. kVp can be lowered to reduce scatter, but this also causes which of the following?
   a. Reduced density
   b. More penumbra
   c. Smaller field size
   d. All of the above
   e. None of the above

4. Aperture diaphragms have what shape?
   a. Round
   b. Square
   c. Rectangular
   d. All of the above
   e. None of the above

5. Limitations of aperture diaphragms include which of the following?
   a. They cause unsharpness.
   b. They allow off-focus radiation to reach the film.
   c. They do not provide light to guide positioning.
   d. All of the above are true.
   e. None of the above is true.

6. The basic parts of a collimator are which of the following?
   a. Light source, mirror, and shutters
   b. Light source, shutters, and lead blockers
   c. Light source, aperture diaphragm, and lead blockers
   d. Light source, mirror, and aperture diaphragm

7. The second-stage shutters (farther from the tube) reduce which of the following?
   a. Off-focus radiation
   b. Unsharpness
   c. Low-energy x-rays
   d. All of the above
   e. None of the above

8. What does the mirror inside the collimator do?
   a. Focuses the x-ray beam
   b. Redirects the x-ray beam to the proper field
   c. Reflects the light beam to the same area as the radiation beam
   d. Redirects the light beam so the tube can be better seen

9. The position of the central ray is determined by which of the following?
   a. The collimator's cross hairs
   b. Measuring downward from the x-ray tube
   c. The red dot projected from the collimator
   d. None of the above

10. Which of the following is true of a positive beam limitation device (PBL)?
    a. It is required on all new fixed radiographic equipment.
    b. It ensures the field size is never larger than the image receptor.
    c. It works automatically to determine film size being used.
    d. All of the above are true.
    e. None of the above is true.

11. Which statement is true about how a radiologic technologist can control a collimator?
    a. One set of shutters can be moved to control the width of the field.
    b. One set of shutters can be moved to control the length of the field.
    c. Both sets of shutters can be moved to control both width and length.
    d. Some equipment allows controlling both sets of shutters, and others allow control of only one.

12. Compensating filters compensate for which of the following?
    a. Uneven rates at which body parts absorb x-rays
    b. The broad spectrum of x-ray photon energy levels in the beam
    c. Using different field sizes
    d. The anode heel effect

13. "Inherent filtration" refers to which of the following?
    a. Compensating filters
    b. Aluminum filters added in the beam
    c. Wedge filters
    d. All of the above
    e. None of the above

14. "Aluminum equivalency" refers to which of the following?
    a. The amount of filtering
    b. The density of a body structure
    c. Materials used in collimator shutters
    d. The x-ray tube housing

15. Which of the following are compensating filters?
    a. Wedge filters
    b. Trough filters
    c. Step-wedge filters
    d. All of the above
    e. None of the above

Answer Key

Answers to Pretest

1. d

2. b

3. d

4. d

5. a

6. d

7. c

8. c

9. a

10. d

Answers to Review

1. Scatter, fog, decreasing, limiting (or restricting)

2. More, compression

3. Higher, image receptor (or film), increased, increased

4. Diaphragms, lead, port of x-ray tube (or housing), smaller

5. Unsharpness (or blurring), off-focus, collimator

6. Shutters, light, mirror, lead, entrance, unsharpness

7. Localizer, central ray (or beam), cross hairs

8. Positive beam limitation device, film cassette

9. Hardening, low, increasing, image, patient dose

10. Added, aluminum equivalency, half-value

11. Compensating, trough (or step-wedge, bowtie, or conic filters), Plexiglas

Answers to Learning Quiz

1. When a high-energy photon comes near an electron in an outer shell, it might undergo the Compton effect. In this case the photon is deflected from its path into a new direction and loses some energy. This low-energy photon is called scatter radiation.

2. Scatter is reduced in thinner body areas or tissues. Two common examples of how tissue can be compressed to reduce scatter are (1) having a patient lie down rather than stand for an abdominal exam because the abdomen is thinner when lying and (2) the compression of the breast in the mammography unit to reduce the scatter from the thicker part of the breast.

3. Three disadvantages of aperture diaphragms compared to collimators are:
   • They cause more unsharpness around the edges of the image.
   • They allow more off-focus radiation to reach the film.
   • They do not provide a light beam to guide the positioning of the patient.

   In general, they are also not as quick or easy to use as collimators. For all these reasons aperture diaphragms are not as commonly used in the present.

4. The function of the first pair of shutters, called the entrance shutters, is to control off- focus radiation. Therefore they are close to the tube. The second set, called second-stage shutters, are farther from the tube to better reduce the unsharpness. Both pairs work together to limit the field size.

5.

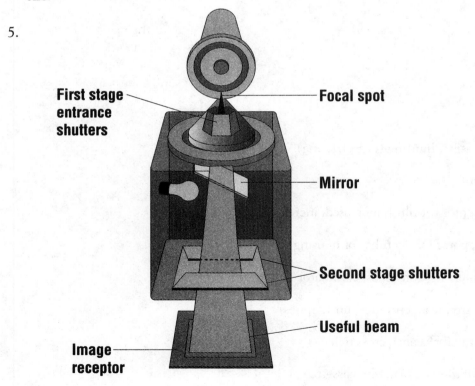

VARIABLE-APERTURE LIGHT-LOCALIZING COLLIMATOR

Your sketch should show the light to one side of the path of the x-ray beam through the collimator. The mirror, positioned at a 45 degree angle in the middle of that path, reflects the light out the collimator in the same position as the x-ray beam.

6. The filtered x-ray beam is said to be "hardened" because the filtering removes much of the low-energy radiation, thereby raising the average energy of the beam. This greater intensity of the beam is, in a sense, "harder."

7. Aluminum offers several advantages as a filtering material. First, as an element it absorbs practical amounts of radiation in sheets that are neither too thick nor too thin. Lead would not make a good filter, for example, because it absorbs too much radiation and would have to be made into an extremely thin layer.

   A second advantage of aluminum is that it is a common element and therefore relatively inexpensive.

   Finally, aluminum is flexible and malleable and can easily be worked into different sizes, shapes, and thicknesses.

   Although other materials such as beryllium and copper are also used in specialized filters, because of its advantages, aluminum has become the standard for filtering.

8. The National Council of Radiation Protection (NCRP) recommends minimum levels of filtration because filtering eliminates much of the low-energy radiation that would not contribute to the image but that would be absorbed in the body, thereby increasing the patient dose.

9. A compensating filter might be used in a chest examination to even out the density of the image if one area was considerably more radiopaque than another. Much fluid or a mass in the lungs on one side, for example, might significantly increase the radiopacity in that area, resulting in less density in the image. Use of a compensating filter on the other side and adjusting exposure factors accordingly would help even out the image.

Answers for Applications

1. Although it is true that lower kVp reduces the amount of scatter, using a low kVp in all circumstances is not the answer because of other effects. With a lower kVp, the mAs selection must be higher to compensate and obtain a diagnostic image, and a higher mAs increases the patient's dose. Contrast also may suffer with lower kVp settings, thus reducing the quality of the image. Therefore the radiologic technologist must seek to balance the goals of reducing scatter and lowering patient dose and obtaining quality images. Higher kVp selections are generally used to best meet these goals.

2. Cones and cylinders are used mainly for head, spine, dental, and gallbladder examinations where very specific small areas are to be imaged.

3. A positive beam limitation device (PBL) works automatically to ensure the field size does not exceed the film size. Sensors, usually built into the examination table or other equipment, gauge the size and position of the film cassette and signal the collimator with this information. The collimator automatically adjusts the field size to be smaller than the cassette and in the right position.

4. A wedge filter might be used with an exam of the foot, for example, to even out the differences in opacity between the heel and toes. The toe area would be filtered more heavily, and exposure factors selected based on the thicker area of the heel, which receives less filtering.

5. The key advantage of lead-impregnated Plexiglas as a filtering material is that it allows light to pass through it, unlike aluminum or other types of filters. Therefore the light localizing system of the collimator can still be used.

Technique Formation

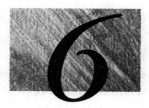

Self-Assessment Pretest

Use this pretest to assess your knowledge of the material in this module before you begin to work through the following exercises. Circle the best answer for each of the following questions. The answers are at the end of this module.

1. Technique charts are designed to do which of the following?
    a. Provide exposure settings for standard exams
    b. Produce high-quality images
    c. Ensure consistency in radiographs
    d. All of the above
    e. None of the above

2. The current flowing through the tube filament is measured as which of the following?
    a. kVp
    b. SID
    c. mA
    d. Generator voltage

3. The kVp selection must be high enough to do which of the following?
    a. Ensure adequate x-ray penetration of the body
    b. Allow a short OID
    c. Reduce unsharpness
    d. All of the above
    e. None of the above

4. What does kVp determine?
    a. The current through the x-ray tube filament
    b. The voltage of the power supplied to the equipment
    c. The velocity of the electrons striking the anode
    d. The number of x-rays produced

5. Changing the SID will change which of the following?
   a. The OID
   b. The kVp
   c. The intensity of the beam reaching the film
   d. All of the above
   e. None of the above

6. Subject contrast results from which of the following?
   a. The intensity of the x-ray beam
   b. The amount of radiation absorbed by different parts of the body
   c. The film's ability to register different levels of contrast
   d. All of the above
   e. None of the above

7. Film developer can affect which of the following?
   a. Image contrast
   b. Scatter radiation fog
   c. Shape distortion
   d. Unsharpness

8. Patient considerations for technique include which of the following?
   a. The patient's overall body size
   b. The thickness of the body area being imaged
   c. The types of tissues in the body area being imaged
   d. All of the above
   e. None of the above

9. Technique charts should specify which of the following?
   a. When a grid is used
   b. How to estimate the patient's height
   c. How large to make the OID
   d. All of the above
   e. None of the above

10. Automatic exposure control systems generally have which of the following?
    a. An automatic timer that ends the exposure when the density is optimum
    b. A built-in Geiger counter that adjusts the kVp during the exposure
    c. A moving collimator that continually changes the field size to control scatter
    d. All of the above
    e. None of the above

Key Terms

Before continuing, be sure you can define the following key terms.

Automatic exposure control system: Technique chart and system in which the length of the exposure is determined automatically by sensors that detect when the density is sufficient.

Automatically programmed radiography (APR): Computer-aided technique charts for determining the best exposure selections for a variety of projections of different body areas.

Calipers: A device for measuring patient thickness.

Central ray: The geometric center of the x-ray beam as it exits the tube from the focal spot; the center point from which all other rays spread out as they move farther away from the tube.

Contrast: The differences in density on adjacent areas of the radiograph; see **subject contrast** and **film contrast.**

Density: The overall amount of blackening on a radiograph; also called optical density or radiographic density.

Distortion: A misrepresentation of the size or shape of the part of the body being examined, as a result of geometric factors; see also **size distortion** and **shape distortion.**

Elongation: Shape distortion in which a structure appears to be longer than it actually is.

Exposure guide: Another term for a technique chart.

Exposure variables: Exposure factors that affect the quality of a radiograph, including kVp, mA, exposure time, and SID.

Fifteen percent rule: The principle that a kVp increase of 15% doubles the exposure.

Film contrast: The inherent ability of a radiographic film to record a range of densities.

Fixed kVp technique chart: A technique chart in which the kVp stays the same but different mAs selections are used for patients of different thickness.

Foreshortening: Shape distortion in which a structure appears to be shorter than it actually is.

Grid: A device designed to allow x-rays to be transmitted directly through the patient to the film but to absorb x-rays scattered within the patient before they reach the film.

High kVp technique chart: A technique chart in which the kVp selection is always high (usually over 100 kVp), such as are used with most chest exams because of the variety of tissue densities present.

Intensifying screen: A device that converts x-ray photons to light photons to help create the latent image on the film, thereby reducing the x-ray exposure required.

Inverse square law: The geometric principle that the intensity of radiation is inversely proportional to the square of the distance from the source of the radiation.

mA: Abbreviation for milliamps, the measure of the flow of electrons from the cathode to the anode in an x-ray tube, which is an indirect measurement of the number of x-ray photons produced in the beam.

Magnification: The geometric phenomenon that the image on a radiograph is always somewhat bigger than the object or structure itself because the x-ray beam continues to disperse as it moves from the object to the image receptor.

mAs: Abbreviation for milliamp-seconds, the product of the tube current in mA and the length of the exposure in seconds.

Object-to-image receptor distance (OID): The distance between the object being radiographed and the film or other image receptor.

Pathology, pathological condition: A disease or condition; for radiographers, pathology usually refers to a condition that causes some visible change in a radiograph.

Radiographic technique: The manipulation of exposure factors to obtain the best quality images possible.

Recorded detail: The degree of sharpness of structures recorded in a radiograph.

Shape distortion: The type of distortion in which the image of the body part is shaped differently from the actual structure, due to improper alignment of the x-ray tube, patient, and image receptor.

Size distortion: The type of distortion that results from magnification of the object in the image.

Source-to-image receptor distance (SID): The distance between the x-ray tube and the film or other image receptor.

Subject contrast: The contrast that results from differences in tissue density in the patient.

Technique chart: One of several different types of charts that list standardized exposure factors for standard exams, with variations for different patient thicknesses.

Unsharpness: The area of unsharpness at the edges of structures caused by geometric properties of the x-ray beam coming from the focal spot.

Variable kVp technique chart: A technique chart in which the mAs stays the same but different kVp selections are used for patients of different thickness.

Topical Outline

The following material is covered in this module.

I. Radiographic technique refers to manipulating exposure factors to get the highest quality images.
   A. Quality images protect the patient by minimizing the patient dose that would be incurred with a repeat exam.
   B. mA controls the current flowing through the tube's filament.
      1. With a low mA, the kVp must be higher or the exposure time longer to achieve adequate density on the image.
      2. A higher mA allows for a shorter exposure time but may lead to loss of detail because of increased focal spot size.
   C. Exposure time determines how long the x-ray beam continues.
      1. Shorter exposure times are beneficial because there is less motion blur.
      2. Often a short exposure time with a high mA produces the most effective mAs.
      3. High-speed screen-film combinations allow for shorter exposure times.
   D. kVp is the most important exposure factor because of its many effects.
      1. kVp determines the velocity of the electrons striking the anode and thus the energy level of the x-rays produced in the beam.
      2. kVp must be high enough to penetrate the body sufficiently to produce enough density on the image; low-energy x-rays are absorbed in the body but do not contribute to the image.
      3. Increasing the kVp 15% doubles the density.
      4. Whereas increasing the mAs to produce more x-ray photons increases the patient dose, increasing the kVp decreases the dose because more x-rays penetrate the body to reach the image receptor rather than being absorbed by the body.
      5. Higher kVp causes more scatter to exit the patient; overall scatter may be reduced by collimation and when appropriate by use of a grid.
      6. Higher kVp also lowers the contrast on the image.
   E. SID is an important exposure factor because it determines the intensity of the x-ray beam.
      1. The inverse square law applies to SID, meaning that doubling the SID causes the intensity of the beam to be one-fourth.
      2. SID is usually standardized at an effective distance for most exams.
II. Image quality factors include density, contrast, recorded detail, and distortion.
   A. Density is the overall blackening on an image.
      1. A good radiograph shows a variation of densities to clearly distinguish the different tissues in the area examined.
   B. Contrast is a combination of subject and film contrast.

1. Subject contrast is produced on the image by the variable absorption rates of the different tissues in the areas being imaged.
2. Film contrast refers to the sensitivity of an x-ray film to show a range of different densities.
3. Higher kVp settings produce more scatter, which causes fog on the image that lowers contrast.

C. Recorded detail is the degree of sharpness of structures recorded in a radiograph.
   1. Patient motion causes blur that decreases detail.
   2. Visible detail depends on good density and contrast.
   3. Detail is better with a small OID, a smaller focal spot, a slower intensifying screen, and a longer SID.

D. Distortion includes magnification and shape distortion.
   1. Magnification is less with a longer SID and a shorter OID.
   2. Shape distortion is minimized by aligning the x-ray beam, the body part being examined, and the image receptor.

III. Patient considerations in radiographic technique include the patient's size, the tissues being examined, the pathological condition, and positioning.

A. Patient thickness affects how many x-rays are absorbed in the body.
   1. Either the kVp or mAs must be increased to compensate for thicker patient areas.
   2. Patient thickness is measured using callipers.
   3. Thicker patients and body parts produce more scatter radiation.

B. kVp and mAs selections depend on the tissues being examined and the variations in tissue density in the body area.

C. Correct patient positioning is necessary to minimize distortion.

IV. Technique charts establish suggested settings for exposure for a particular exam with the equipment used in the department.

A. Technique charts are established by radiologists, radiographers, and medical physicists in the department, using the specific equipment present for specific types of standard exams.

B. Radiologic technologists consult technique charts to determine the best exposure factors for a given patient for a standard exam.

C. Technique charts protect the patient because they minimize the need for repeat exams.

D. The technique chart states whether and when to use grids, different screen-film combinations, and the kVp and mAs selections for different patient thicknesses.

E. There are four standard types of technique charts.
   1. The variable-kVp chart uses a standard mAs and a variable kVp setting based on the patient's thickness.
      a. Contrast may vary with a variable kVp chart.
      b. Exposure changes are easy to make to compensate for different body sizes.
      c. Calipers are used to accurately measure body thickness.
   2. The fixed kVp system uses one kVp setting and varies the mAs depending on the body thickness.
      a. Contrast and density are more consistent.
      b. Exposure time is shorter.
      c. More scatter is produced, lowering overall contrast.
   3. The high kVp technique keeps the kVp high (over 100 kVp) for all studies and is typically used for chest exams.
   4. The automatic exposure control system has an electronic timer that ends the exposure as soon as there is optimum density on the image.

F. Anatomically programmed radiography uses a computerized system to guide exposure selections based on the desired projection and the patient's size.

Review

1. _____, also called exposure guides, provide standardized exposure selections for routine exams. Using these charts _____ the chances of having to perform a repeat exam.

2. Because mA controls the current flow through the tube's _____, increasing the mA will increase the number of x-rays produced. Using a higher mA will allow using a faster _____ to produce the same mAs. This shorter time reduces the risk of blur caused by _____. Using a(n) _____ screen-film combination will also reduce the exposure time.

3. _____ is the most important exposure factor because it affects so many other things. With a higher kVp, for example, _____ scatter radiation is produced. More x-rays also penetrate the body, producing _____ density on the image. In fact, increasing the kVp by only _____ will double the density. There needs to be a balance between kVp and _____, however, because as one is raised, the other generally must be lowered.

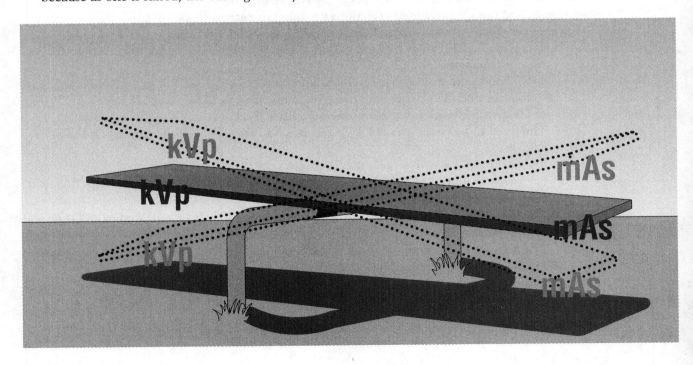

4. Use of _____ and _____ will help reduce scatter reaching the image receptor when a higher kVp is used. The kVp can also be lowered, but in that case the patient dose is generally _____.

5. The _____ law refers to the diminishing of the intensity of the x-ray beam as it spreads out from the tube. This is why the exposure factor selections must be adjusted when the _____ is changed. Doubling the SID cuts the beam's intensity to _____ of what it was.

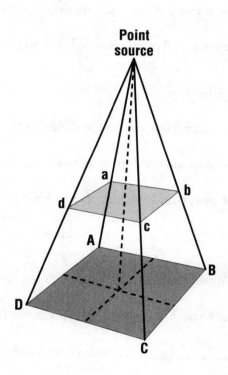

6. _____ is the overall blackening on the image, produced by x-rays penetrating the body and reaching the image receptor. Too many x-rays would turn the film completely _____, and if there were too few the film would look _____. The ideal image has a range of densities, called _____. Fog caused by scatter radiation at higher kVp levels _____ contrast.

7. The form of distortion called _____ is present in all radiographs but is lower if the OID is _____. Shape distortion, the other kind of distortion, can be minimized if the central ray is well aligned with the body area and the _____.

8. The _____ the patient or body part, the higher must be exposure factors. Also, thicker body areas produce more _____ radiation. Measuring patient thickness with _____ is therefore an important aspect of many exams.

9. Technique charts are created in the department by _____ and _____ to use with the specific equipment present in the department. A technique chart gives the standardized settings for different exams, and often you need only to choose the right selections for a given patient's _____.

10. With a(n) _____ - _____ chart, the mAs is the same and the kVp selection changes depending on the body area being imaged and the patient's _____. An advantage of this kind of chart is that it is easy to make small exposure changes, but a disadvantage is that increasing the kVp can reduce _____ on the image.

11. To measure the patient with calipers, measure either through the central ray's _____ and _____ points, or through the _____ part of the body part, depending on what is specified by the technique _____. Every radiologic technologist should measure patients in the same way.

12. An advantage of the _____-kVp system, in which only the _____ is modified depending on patient thickness, is lower patient dose and _____ exposure time. A disadvantage is that more _____ may result and cause fog on the image.

13. A high kVp chart uses a kVp in the range of _____. This is used typically for _____ exams.

14. Automatic exposure control systems have a(n) _____ that ends the exposure when optimum density is obtained. Standard selections are typically used for _____ and _____. Even with automatic systems it is important to _____ the patient properly to determine thickness and to _____ the body part perfectly over the timing device sensors.

15. Using a system of anatomically programmed radiography, the computer helps you make selections by offering a choice of various _____ for the body area. As with other systems, exposure selections are _____ depending on patient size.

Learning Quiz

The following material includes interactive exercises found in the CD-ROM version of this module operated in the "Student Mode." These questions will allow you to review the concepts presented in this module and will help you gain a more complete understanding of the material.

1. Explain at least two advantages of using technique charts.

2. Why is a short exposure time with a higher mA generally better than a longer exposure time with a lower mA — if the mAs is the same in both instances?

3. The 15% rule means that increasing kVp will double the density. Leaving the kVp unchanged but doing what to the mAs will also double the density?

4. Sometimes it is necessary to use a higher kVp to penetrate the body area sufficiently to obtain a good image. What can be done to minimize the effects of the scatter radiation produced at higher kVp levels?

5. How does patient motion affect the level of recorded detail? What can the radiologic technologist do to prevent this loss of image quality?

6. Describe the proper positioning of the central ray, patient, and image receptor for the least amount of distortion. Also, what OID is ideal?

7. Why is it important to check and calibrate the mA, kVp, and timer settings before developing technique charts for radiographic equipment?

8. Describe how a patient is measured with calipers.

9. Name the primary advantage and disadvantage of the variable-kVp technique chart.

10. Name at least two advantages and disadvantages of the fixed-kVp technique chart.

Applications

1. Describe the balance between kVp and mAs when making exposure selections, listing the disadvantages of having either factor set too high or too low.

2. Give an example when a high-contrast film might be used, and explain why.

3. Give an example of when a low kVp would be used, and an example of when a high kVp would be used.

4. With a fixed-kVp chart designed for small, average, and large patients, how much would you increase the average mAs for a large patient? How much would you decrease it for a small patient?

5. What kind of technique would generally be used for barium studies?

Posttest

Circle the best answer for each of the following questions. Your instructor has the correct answers.

1. Using technique charts helps ensure which of the following?
   a. Patients receive minimal radiation
   b. Equipment receives routine maintenance
   c. Chemicals are periodically changed in the developer
   d. All of the above
   e. None of the above

2. Control panel selections allow determination of which of the following?
   a. How many x-rays reach the patient
   b. The energy level of the x-rays
   c. The length of time the x-ray beam is on
   d. All of the above
   e. None of the above

3. In general, which is better?
   a. A longer exposure time
   b. A shorter exposure time
   c. An exposure time standardized for all exams
   d. Any exposure time is fine

4. kVp affects which of the following?
   a. Contrast in the image
   b. The amount of scatter radiation produced
   c. Patient dose
   d. All of the above
   e. None of the above

5. Increasing the kVp by 15% does which of the following?
   a. Doubles the density on the film
   b. Halves the density on the film
   c. Has no effect on density but doubles the contrast
   d. None of the above

6. When high kVp technique is used, which of the following is true?
   a. Collimation is needed to reduce scatter.
   b. A grid may be needed to absorb some of the scatter.
   c. Contrast is reduced.
   d. All of the above are true.
   e. None of the above is true.

7. The radiologic technologist applies the inverse square law to which of the following?
   a. Distance from cathode to anode
   b. Object-to-image receptor distance
   c. Source-to-image receptor distance
   d. All of the above
   e. None of the above

8. Image quality factors include which of the following?
   a. Density
   b. Contrast
   c. Detail
   d. All of the above
   e. None of the above

9. A high-contrast film is generally used for which of the following?
   a. Larger patients
   b. Smaller patients
   c. Body areas with large variations in absorption rates
   d. Body areas with small variations in absorption rates

10. For the best result, the central ray should be which of the following?
    a. Perpendicular to the image receptor
    b. Perpendicular to the part being imaged
    c. Positioned in the center of the area being imaged
    d. All of the above
    e. None of the above

11. Technique charts are established based on which of the following?
   a. Small patients
   b. Large patients
   c. Specific x-ray equipment
   d. An average of all the equipment in the department

12. Technique charts take into account which of the following?
   a. kVp
   b. The x-ray equipment
   c. Screen-film combinations
   d. All of the above
   e. None of the above

13. Why do technique charts help reduce patient dose?
   a. Because kVp is always kept low
   b. Because mAs is always kept low
   c. Because the need for repeated exams is minimal
   d. Because faster screen-film combinations are used

14. Technique charts are created by which of the following?
   a. The equipment manufacturer
   b. Radiologists and technologists in the department
   c. The authors of radiographic textbooks
   d. Darkroom technicians

15. With a variable kVp chart, the kVp for a particular exam is selected based on which of the following?
   a. The patient's thickness
   b. The patient's ability to hold still
   c. The patient's age
   d. The varying mAs setting

Answer Key

Answers to Pretest

1. d

2. c

3. a

4. c

5. c

6. b

7. a

8. d

9. a

10. a

Answers to Review

1. Technique charts, minimize

2. Filament, exposure time, patient motion, high-speed

3. kVp, more, greater (or more), 15%, mAs

4. Grids, collimator, higher

5. Inverse square, SID, one-fourth

6. Density, black, white (or clear), contrast, diminishes (decreases, lowers)

7. Magnification (size distortion), short, image receptor (film)

8. Thicker, scatter, calipers

9. Radiologists, medical physicists, thickness

10. Variable-kVp, thickness, contrast

11. Entrance, exit, thickest, chart

12. Fixed, mAs, shorter, scatter

13. 100-120 kVp, chest

14. Electronic timer, kVp, mA, measure, position

15. Projections, modified (or selected)

Answers to Learning Quiz

1. Technique charts standardize the exposure selections to obtain the best possible image on the particular equipment being used and therefore minimize the chance of error. This also protects the patient because it reduces the risk of having to do a repeat examination, which would increase patient dose.

2. As long as the combination of mA and time is the same in both instances, the mAs is the same and has the same effect on the image. The advantage of the shorter exposure time is that the risk of blur due to patient motion is lower.

3. Doubling the mAs will double the density. Therefore doubling the mAs has the same effect on density as increasing the kVp by 15%.

4. Scatter can be reduced with the use of a grid when appropriate and in all cases by using collimation to narrow the area receiving radiation.

5. Patient motion causes blur, which is a loss of recorded detail. Shorter exposure times can help minimize the effect of patient motion, and helping the patient remain motionless can help prevent motion.

6. To minimize shape distortion, the central ray should be perpendicular to the body part and the image receptor and be centered on the area being imaged. The OID should be as short as possible to minimize magnification.

7. Technique charts will guide the use of the radiographic equipment for many future examinations, and therefore it is important that the controls function properly and are set within acceptable limits. In this way, the settings provided by the technique chart will produce the best possible images and minimize patient dose. The mA, kVp, and timer settings must all be checked and calibrated.

8. Calipers are used to measure patient thickness for an examination. Measurements are taken at one of two places: either the thickest part of the body area being imaged, or from the entrance to the exit point of the central ray. The method used is standardized within the department and used consistently.

9. The primary advantage of the variable-kVp chart is that small exposure changes are easily made to compensate for differences in body size. The primary disadvantage is that with higher kVp selections, the contrast is low.

10. The advantages of the fixed-kVp chart are that the mAs is lowered to compensate for smaller body sizes, thus decreasing patient dose; density and contrast are usually consistent; and exposure time is generally lower. Disadvantages are that more scatter is produced, lowering contrast, and it may be more difficult to use the mAs settings to compensate for small changes in body size.

Answers for Applications

1. In general, the higher the kVp, the lower the mAs and vice versa. However, the relationship is not that simple. If the kVp is too low, the x-rays will not have enough energy to penetrate the body regardless of how many x-rays there are (with higher mAs). If the kVp is too high, too much scatter will be produced, even if the mAs is set low to prevent too many x-rays from reaching the image receptor and making the image too dense. If the mAs is too low, not enough x-rays may be produced to penetrate the body to create an image, and if the mAs is too high, the patient dose may be increased and too many x-rays may penetrate the body and cause too much density.

2. A high-contrast film is used when there is not much variation in tissue densities in the body area being imaged. Because the resulting radiograph otherwise would not show much contrast or variation in the densities of adjacent areas on the image, use of a high-contrast film will help bring out more subtle differences in tissues. Mammography, exams of breast tissue, is a good example of the use of high-contrast film.

3. A low kVp is used for thinner body areas, such as in mammography or the examination of a hand or foot. A high kVp is used for a thicker area with denser tissues, such as a chest examination.

4. For a large patient, mAs would typically be increased 50%. For a small patient, it would be decreased by 50%.

5. A high kVp technique is often used for barium studies to ensure the x-ray penetration of the body area is sufficient to produce a good image, given that the barium-filled areas will appear more dense.

Exposure Selection

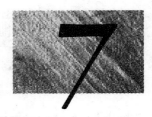

Self-Assessment Pretest

Use this pretest to assess your knowledge of the material in this module before you begin to work through the following exercises. Circle the best answer for each of the following questions. The answers are at the end of this module.

1. What do areas of high density on a radiograph indicate?
   a. More x-rays exiting from the patient
   b. Fewer x-rays exiting from the patient
   c. Poor selection of exposure factors
   d. That the development solution should be changed

2. Higher kVp selections generally do which of the following?
   a. Penetrate the body poorly
   b. Require higher mAs selections
   c. Cause more scatter radiation
   d. All of the above
   e. None of the above

3. What is a good starting point for determining the recommended kVp for a particular exam?
   a. The department's technique chart
   b. The patient's weight
   c. The x-ray equipment's tube rating chart
   d. Any of the above

4. Changing the mA setting from 100 to 200 causes what change?
   a. The number of x-rays in the beam doubles.
   b. The number of x-rays in the beam is cut in half.
   c. The energy level of x-rays in the beam doubles.
   d. The energy level of x-rays in the beam is cut in half.

5. How is mAs calculated?
   a. Milliamperes plus seconds
   b. Milliamperes divided by seconds
   c. Milliamperes times seconds
   d. None of the above

6. Increasing the SID generally does which of the following?
   a. Decreases magnification
   b. Increases magnification
   c. Has no effect on magnification
   d. Answer depends on other variables

7. Why is an SID over 72 inches seldom used?
   a. It is impossible.
   b. It is impractical.
   c. It causes too much magnification.
   d. Too much scatter results.

8. Which of the following is true?
   a. The larger the focal spot, the higher the technique capacity.
   b. The larger the focal spot, the greater the penumbra.
   c. The larger the focal spot, the higher mAs settings that are possible.
   d. All of the above are true.
   e. None of the above is true.

9. What is the disadvantage of using a grid?
   a. Poor contrast
   b. Longer exposures and potential motion blur
   c. Larger penumbra
   d. Increased patient radiation dose

10. How is filtration measured?
    a. mm C+ equivalent
    b. mm H_2O equivalent
    c. mm Al equivalent
    d. mm Ph equivalent

Key Terms

Before continuing, be sure you can define the following key terms.

Added filtration: Aluminum filters added outside the tube to increase filtration of the primary beam.

Aluminum equivalency: A measurement of the filtering capacity of a filter comparing it to the filtration provided by aluminum.

Collimator: A device, usually adjustable, that restricts the size of the x-ray beam as it emerges from the tube.

Compensating filter: A type of added filter designed to compensate for different tissue densities in different body areas by filtering the beam through one area more than through another.

Contrast: The differences in density on adjacent areas of the radiograph.

Contrast medium: A radiopaque substance injected or ingested into the body for improved visualization of structures in a radiographic or fluoroscopic examination.

Contrast improvement factor: A measure of how much contrast improves in a radiograph by using a grid.

Density: The overall amount of blackening on a radiograph; also called optical density or radiographic density.

Filter: A device, usually made of aluminum, inserted into the path of the x-ray beam near the tube to absorb the low-energy (long-wavelength) x-rays, thereby increasing the average energy of the beam; see **inherent filtration** and **added filtration.**

Focal spot: The area of the anode where x-ray photons are produced by bombardment of electrons from the cathode.

Generator: The electrical device that produces the high-voltage current necessary for the x-ray tube.

Grid: A device designed to allow x-rays to be transmitted directly through the patient to the film but to absorb x-rays scattered within the patient before they reach the film.

Grid ratio: The ratio between the height of the lead strips in a grid and the width of the interspace material between them.

Hardening: Refers to the use of filtration to remove low-energy x-rays from the beam and thereby raise the average energy level.

Inherent filtration: The tube elements that filter the beam, including the glass envelope and the insulating oil.

Intensifying screen: A device that converts x-ray photons to light photons to help create the latent image on the film, thereby reducing the x-ray exposure required.

Inverse square law: The geometric principle that the intensity of radiation is inversely proportional to the square of the distance from the source of the radiation.

kVp: The abbreviation for kilovolt peak, a measure of the electrical potential between the cathode and anode of the x-ray tube, which determines the energy level of the x-rays in the beam.

mA: Abbreviation for milliamps, the measure of the flow of electrons from the cathode to the anode in an x-ray tube, which is an indirect measurement of the number of x-ray photons produced in the beam.

mAs: Abbreviation for milliamp-seconds, the product of the tube current in mA and the length of the exposure in seconds.

Magnification: The geometric phenomenon that the image on a radiograph is always somewhat bigger than the object or structure itself because the x-ray beam continues to disperse as it moves from the object to the image receptor.

Object-to-image receptor distance (OID): The distance between the object being radiographed and the film or other image receptor.

Quality: Referring to the x-ray beam, quality is the average energy level of the x-rays in the beam, determined by the kVp selection.

Quantity: Referring to the x-ray beam, quantity is a measure of how many x-rays are in the beam, determined by the mAs selection.

Recorded detail: The degree of sharpness of structures recorded in a radiograph.

Ripple factor: A rating measure for generators, referring to how much the voltage drops from the maximum; single-phase power, for example, has a higher ripple than three-phase power.

Scatter radiation: X-rays produced inside the patient's body or another substance when x-ray photons within the primary beam interact with atoms in that substance to produce Compton or classical scattering of x-ray photons in different directions.

Source-to-image receptor distance (SID): The distance between the x-ray tube and the film or other image receptor.

Technique chart: One of several different types of charts that list standardized exposure factors for standard exams, with variations for different patient thicknesses.

Unsharpness: The area of unsharpness at the edges of structures caused by geometric properties of the x-ray beam coming from the focal spot.

Topical Outline

The following material is covered in this module.

I. Primary technique factors — kVp and mAs — affect exposure selection and determine levels of density and contrast.
   A. High-density areas indicate more x-rays exiting the patient; low-density areas indicate fewer x-rays exiting the patient.
   B. The perfect balance of high and low densities, or contrast, depends on the right combination of exposure factors.
      1. Technique charts guide exposures but do not replace the need for knowledge of the effects of all variables and judgments about how the variables interact.
   C. The kVp determines the quality, or energy level, of the x-ray beam.
      1. At higher kVp levels, there is more penetration of the patient, resulting in higher density.
      2. Higher kVp levels reduce patient exposure caused by the absorption of lower-energy x-rays.
      3. Higher kVp levels cause more scatter radiation, however, reducing contrast.
      4. Selection of the appropriate kVp involves considerations of the thickness of the part being examined, the use of a grid to reduce scatter, the screen-film combination, and the use of any contrast media.
   D. The mAs determines the quantity of photons in the x-ray beam.
      1. The number of x-ray photons produced is directly proportional to the filament current, measured in mA.
      2. mAs, or the mA multiplied by the exposure time, determines the total number of x-ray photons during an exposure.
      3. The exposure time is usually kept as short as possible to minimize the chance of motion blur.
      4. With some radiographic equipment you can select the mA and the exposure time separately, whereas with falling load generators you may be able to select only the mAs, and the equipment will determine the precise mA and time factors.
      5. Density in the radiograph is directly proportional to the mAs; doubling the mAs doubles the density.
II. Secondary factors also affect exposure selection.
   A. SID is an important consideration because the x-ray beam spreads out as it travels from the tube.
      1. Following the inverse square law, doubling the SID produces one fourth as much density on the radiograph.
      2. SID is standardized, usually at 40 or 72 inches, to balance practicality with good detail and acceptable levels of magnification.
      3. SID is determined by the technique chart; when SID is increased, increase the mAs to compensate.
      4. SID might be altered because of other equipment in place around a patient or because an extremely large patient needs more penetrating energy.
   B. OID is usually kept as short as possible because a larger OID increases magnification and penumbra, reducing the amount of detail.
   C. Choice of focal spot size is another important determination.
      1. Smaller focal spots result in less unsharpness and produce greater detail, but more heat is produced in the anode and therefore higher energy levels are limited.

2. Larger focal spots result in more unsharpness and thus less detail but can be used with higher-energy technique.

3. Small focal spots are generally used for examining thinner parts of the body, and larger focal spots for more dense or thicker areas or when very high technique factors are required.

D. A grid may be used with higher kVp selections to absorb up to 90% of the scatter.

1. The grid is made of strips of radiopaque material, such as lead, separated by radiolucent material that lets x-rays pass through only when they are in a straight line from the tube to the image receptor.

2. The contrast improvement factor measures how much better contrast is in the image when a grid is used.

3. The disadvantage of grids is that the exposure must be increased to penetrate the grid, resulting in increased patient exposure.

E. Intensifying screens are used in combination with the film in most radiographic procedures because the fluorescent light produced by the screen helps expose the film, allowing for a lower radiation dose to the patient.

III. Filtration also affects exposure selection.

A. Filtration includes inherent filtration and added filtration.

B. The benefit of added filtration is the absorption of low-energy x-rays that could add nothing to the image but would be absorbed in the body, increasing the patient dose.

C. Compensating filters are used to even out density when wide differences in body tissues or density would cause too much variation in density on the finished radiograph.

IV. The radiographic equipment's generator is a final factor affecting exposure.

A. A falling load generator allows for selecting only mAs, and the equipment selects the optimal mA and time exposure.

B. Ripple factor, the difference between the maximum voltage and the lowest level to which it falls, causes fluctuation in the x-ray beam.

C. Three-phase power generators produce a more consistent beam than the original single-phase generators, but modern high-frequency generators are still better and provide a ripple factor less than 1%.

Review

1. Areas of _____ tissue density appear dark on a radiograph. The difference between areas of high and low density is called _____. Both density and contrast are affected by the two primary exposure selections, _____ and _____, as well as other factors.

2. mAs controls the quantity of the x-ray beam, while kVp controls the _____ of the beam. Higher kVp settings penetrate the body better, producing more _____ in the image, but higher kVp selections also cause more _____ radiation to be produced. Scatter reduces the _____ in the image.

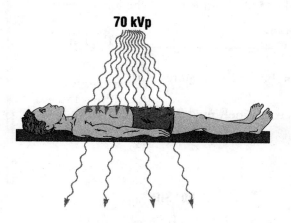

At lower kVp, the beam's penetrating ability is lower.

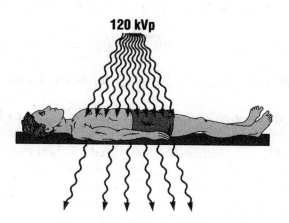

Increased kVp increases the efficiency of the beam.

3. Use of higher kVp selections usually means the _____ selection can be lower. kVp selection is affected by other variables too, however, such as the use of a(n) _____, which requires a higher kVp selection, as well as the exact _____-screen combination used.

4. A(n) _____ time exposure helps prevent motion blur. To achieve the same mAs with a shorter time exposure, the mA selection can be _____. If you need to double the density on the radiograph, double the _____ selection.

5. The source-to-image receptor distance, or _____, is related to magnification. The longer the SID, the _____ the magnification. Because of the _____ law, the longer the SID, the _____ intense is the beam. Therefore a shorter SID requires a(n) _____ mAs selection to compensate. An SID of _____ inches is routinely used for many exams, and an SID of _____ inches is typically used for chest exams.

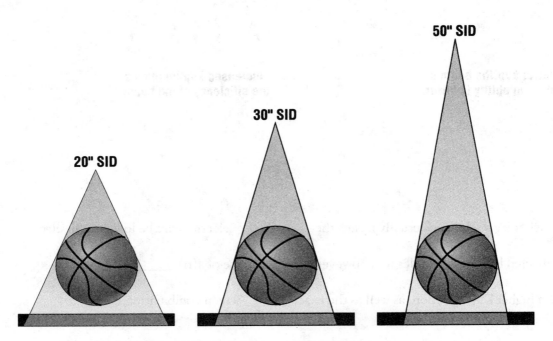

Magnification decreases as SID increases and increases as SID decreases.

6. The OID should generally be kept as _____ as possible because longer OIDs cause more

_____, which diminishes detail.

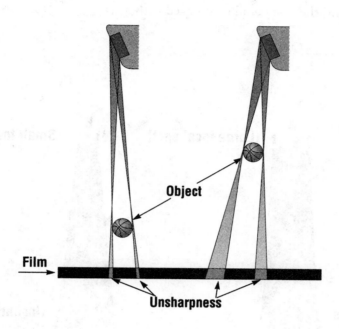

7. Using a(n) _____ focal spot size decreases unsharpness and therefore improves recorded _____. At higher energy levels, however, using a small focal spot could cause the _____ to overheat. The effect of increased blurring is to cause _____ on the radiograph. Ideally, the best detail is achieved with a(n) _____ focal spot, a(n) _____ SID, and a(n) _____ OID.

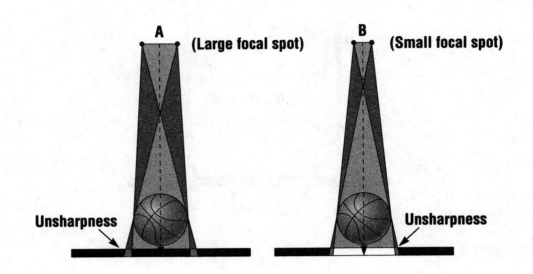

8. A grid is composed of strips of _____ material such as lead, which do not let radiation through, separated by radiolucent material that lets x-rays in a straight line from the tube to the image receptor pass through. The lead strips absorb x-rays not traveling in a straight line, such as _____ radiation. When using a grid, a(n) _____ kVp selection is necessary.

9. The contrast _____ factor measures how much the use of a grid improves the contrast in an image. A factor of 2, for example, would mean there is _____ as much contrast using the grid. Grids can absorb up to _____% of scatter radiation.

10. The use of intensifying screens _____ the patient radiation dose. Most exams use screens for this reason, although their use produces shorter _____ scales.

11. _____ filtration is caused by the equipment itself, such as the tube's glass envelope, whereas _____ filtration is intentionally used to filter the x-ray beam. Removing the low-energy photons, called _____ the beam, also reduces the patient radiation dose because these low-energy photons add nothing to the image but are _____ in the body. Another type of filter, called a(n) _____ filter, is used to even out the density on the image when there are significant differences in tissue density or thickness.

12. The _____ factor is a measure of the drop in voltage from the peak voltage. Three-phase power has much less ripple than the old _____ power, although high-frequency generators today have less than 1% ripple.

Learning Quiz

The following material includes interactive exercises found in the CD-ROM version of this module operated in the "Student Mode." These questions will allow you to review the concepts presented in this module and will help you gain a more complete understanding of the material.

1. Explain the effects of the following variables on density, contrast, and recorded detail:

kVp

mAs

Focal spot size

SID

Grid use

2. Explain the difference between the kVp and mAs selections in terms of the quality and quantity of the x-ray beam.

3. Explain why magnification occurs in any radiograph. Explain the effect of long or short SIDs on magnification. Finally, what is the effect of OID on magnification? Make a simple sketch here showing the x-ray tube, the beam, the patient, and the image receptor, and label the SID and OID. (Hint: The way you sketch the x-ray beam should illustrate the principle of magnification.)

4. Unsharpness reduces the amount of detail on the radiograph. Explain how both SID and focal spot size affect unsharpness.

5. Draw a simple sketch that shows how a grid absorbs scatter radiation. Show the lead strips in your grid and the path of x-rays from the tube through the grid. Also show how an x-ray reaching the grid from a different angle (as would occur with scatter) cannot pass through it.

6. Explain how using an intensifying screen allows for an exposure with a lower radiation dose to the patient.

7. Why is a minimum of added filtration used in all examinations?

Applications

1. The technique chart for a particular exam calls for an mAs selection of 100. At an exposure time of 0.5 seconds, what is the mA setting?

2. For a given kVp selection that is enough to penetrate the body part and result in some density at an mAs selection of 50, what effect on density will occur from an mAs selection of 150?

3. The technique chart calls for an SID of 40 inches, a kVp of 100, and an mAs of 80. Because there is equipment in the way that cannot be moved, you are forced to use an SID of 20 inches. Keeping the kVp the same, what mAs should you use?

4. Because of a pathological condition, a patient's left lung has become much more dense than the right lung. The radiologist requests that you use a compensating filter to even out the density between the two sides. You choose to use a wedge filter. Which side of the body do you expose through the thicker side of the filter? Explain why.

Posttest

Circle the best answer for each of the following questions. Your instructor has the correct answers.

1. What does kVp selection determine?
   a. The quantity of x-rays in the beam
   b. The quality of x-rays in the beam
   c. The exposure time
   d. All of the above
   e. None of the above

2. Factors that affect the kVp selection may include which of the following?
   a. Tissue thickness
   b. Use of a grid
   c. Use of contrast media
   d. All of the above
   e. None of the above

3. Which of the following is true?
   a. The more electrons that pass from the cathode to the anode, the more x-rays are produced.
   b. The more electrons that pass from the cathode to the anode, the higher the mAs setting.
   c. The more electrons that pass from the cathode to the anode, the higher the quantity of the x-ray beam.
   d. All of the above are true.
   e. None of the above is true.

4. Reducing the exposure time also helps reduce which of the following?
   a. Patient exposure
   b. Motion blur
   c. Both of the above
   d. Neither of the above

5. Because of the inverse square law, how is density on a radiography affected if the SID is doubled?
   a. Density is doubled.
   b. Density is halved.
   c. Density is four times as much.
   d. Density is one fourth as much.

6. If you are using a longer SID than that listed in the technique chart, what should you do to maintain good density?
   a. Decrease the kVp
   b. Increase the OID
   c. Use a grid
   d. Increase the mAs

7. If you double the SID from that listed in the technique chart, how much should you change the mAs to have the same level of density?
   a. Set the mAs twice as high
   b. Set the mAs four times as high
   c. Set the mAs half as high
   d. Set the mAs one fourth as high

8. In what situation might you have to use an SID shorter than that given in the technique chart?
   a. With a very thin patient
   b. When equipment interferes with positioning
   c. When the x-ray tube is overheating
   d. When children are fidgety

9. A larger OID has what effect on unsharpness?
   a. Increased unsharpness
   b. Decreased unsharpness
   c. No effect on unsharpness
   d. Effect depends on kVp

10. What is the main reason small focal spots cannot always be used?
   a. The generator could not consistently supply enough power.
   b. Patient exposure would be too great in some circumstances.
   c. Grids cannot be used with small focal spots.
   d. The x-ray tube would overheat.

11. Grids are used to do which of the following?
   a. Improve density
   b. Reduce magnification
   c. Reduce scatter
   d. Lower patient exposure

12. Which x-rays can pass through a grid?
   a. Those traveling in a straight line
   b. Those deflected in the patient's body
   c. Those scattered inside the patient
   d. Those absorbed inside the patient

13. What does a contrast improvement factor of 2 mean?
   a. Using a grid doubles the amount of contrast on an image.
   b. Using a grid halves the amount of contrast on an image.
   c. Using a grid doubles the density with out changing the contrast.
   d. Using a grid halves the density without changing the contrast.

14. Inherent filtration includes which of the following?
   a. The x-ray tube glass envelope
   b. Aluminum filters mounted in the tube port
   c. Intensifying screens
   d. Grids

15. Why do federal regulations require minimum filtration levels?
   a. To standardize image quality
   b. To protect radiographers
   c. To minimize patient dose
   d. To guard against x-ray tube malfunctions

Answer Key

1. a

2. c

3. a

4. a

5. c

6. a

7. b

8. d

9. d

10. c

Answers to Review

1. Low, contrast, kVp, mAs

2. Quality, density, scatter, contrast

3. mAs, grid, film

4 Shorter, increased, mAs

5. SID, less, inverse square, less, lower, 40, 72

6. Short, unsharpness (or magnification)

7. Smaller, detail, x-ray tube (or anode), unsharpness, small, long, short

8. Radiopaque, scatter, higher

9. Improvement, twice, 90

10. Reduces, contrast

11. Inherent, added, hardening, absorbed, compensating

12. Ripple, single-phase

Answers to Learning Quiz

1. kVp must be high enough to penetrate the body part in order to make enough density to provide good recorded detail. If kVp is too high, scatter will result and contrast will be poor and less detail will be present.

   mAs is directly correlated with density and must be high enough to make good density. With the right amount of density, contrast and detail will be good.

   A smaller focal spot size produces better detail. Density and contrast are not related to focal spot size.

   A longer SID produces less unsharpness and thus better detail. With a longer SID, mAs must be increased to compensate to provide enough density. Contrast is not directly related to SID.

   Grid use cuts down on scatter and thus provides better contrast and visibility of detail. Higher kVp is needed to obtain adequate density.

2. The kVp determines the quality of the x-ray beam, which means the energy level of the photons in the beam. High-energy photons penetrate the body better, whereas low-energy photons are often absorbed. mAs determines the quantity of photons in the x-ray beam, or how many x-rays are in the beam to penetrate the body and result in density on the radiograph.

3. Magnification is inevitable in any radiograph because of the inverse square law. The x-ray beam continues to spread out after it passes through the body, making the image on the film somewhat larger than in reality. Because the angle of spread is greater with a short SID, the magnification is greater with a short SID and less with a long SID. Magnification is greater with a large OID because the beam continues to spread out more after leaving the body more when the OID is large.

   Your sketch of this situation should show the x-ray beam spreading out from the tube and continuing to spread out after it passes through the body on the way to the image receptor.

4. Unsharpness is greater with a shorter SID because of the geometric factors involved. A longer SID reduces the unsharpness.

   A smaller focal spot causes less unsharpness because the beam more nearly comes from a point source rather than an area. Unfortunately, because small focal spots may lead to overheating with higher exposure selections, they cannot always be used.

5. Your sketch should look something like the illustration below. Most important is the concept that x-rays traveling in a straight line from the tube can pass through the spaces between the lead strips, whereas x-rays traveling at an angle (those that have been scattered) cannot pass through.

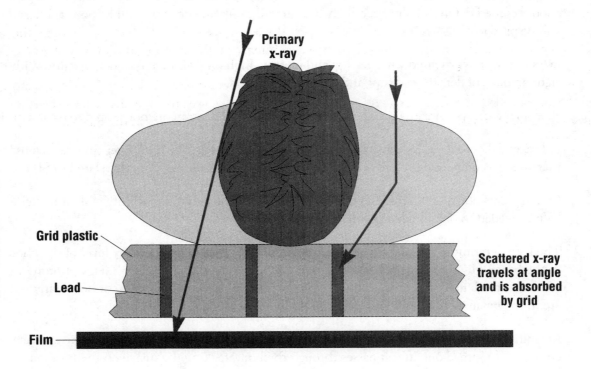

6. When a screen is not used, the film is exposed by x-ray photons only. Because enough photons must reach the film to result in enough density for a good image, the exposure must be more intense. When a screen is used, however, most of the film exposure is caused by the light photons generated when x-ray photons strike the screen. Therefore fewer x-ray photons are needed to make the exposure, and a less intense x-ray beam can be used. Therefore the patient dose is lower.

7. A minimum of added filtration is used in all examinations to absorb the low-energy photons from the beam. These x-rays would contribute nothing to the image but are most likely to be absorbed in the body, thereby increasing the patient's dose. Filtration therefore lowers the patient's dose. Federal regulations require some levels of filtering.

Answers for Applications

1. Remember that mAs equals mA times seconds. To calculate mA, therefore, divide the mAs by the seconds. In this case, the mAs of 100 divided by an exposure time of 0.5 seconds equals an mA setting of 200.

2. Remember that for a given kVp selection that is enough to penetrate the body part and result in some density, the density is directly proportional to the mAs. Therefore, if you triple the mAs as in this example, the density will also triple.

Remember that density is directly proportional to the mAs and that the intensity of the beam is governed by the inverse square law. If the SID is cut in half, its intensity will be four times as great. Therefore you must compensate by selecting an mAs one fourth the original setting to achieve the same density. The new mAs would therefore be 20.

The thicker side of the wedge filter should be positioned over the less dense side of the body, in this case the patient's right lung. Remember that the x-ray beam will be less intense on the thicker side of the wedge filter because more x-ray photons have been filtered out on that side. Fewer x-rays are needed to penetrate the body on that side because the tissue density is less. On the left side, however, where the tissue density is greater, a more intense x-ray beam is needed to penetrate the body. Using the filter in this way, to compensate for density differences in the body, helps ensure that both sides of the radiograph have enough density in the image.

Film Processing

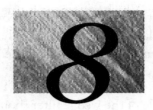

Self-Assessment Pretest

Use this pretest to assess your knowledge of the material in this module before you begin to work through the following exercises. Circle the best answer for each of the following questions. The answers are at the end of this module.

1. Which layer in radiographic film contains silver halide crystals?
   a. The base
   b. The adhesive
   c. The emulsion
   d. The supercoat

2. When can the latent image on a film be seen?
   a. Only after being developed into a manifest image
   b. Immediately after exposure
   c. After being loaded into a computer
   d. All of the above
   e. None of the above

3. Chemical processing converts which of the following?
   a. Free electrons into sensitivity specks
   b. Sensitivity specks into atomic silver
   c. Atomic silver into black silver grains
   d. Positive silver ions into atomic silver

4. What are the four characteristics of a radiographic film?
   a. Speed, contrast, latitude, and color
   b. Contrast, latitude, recorded detail, and intensity
   c. Speed, latitude, recorded detail, and contrast
   d. Contrast, speed, recorded detail, and color

5. Film speed refers to which of the following?
   a. The amount of film blackening resulting from a set exposure
   b. How long it takes for a film to be developed
   c. How long it takes for a film to turn completely black
   d. Double-emulsion film only

6. Which statement is true?
   a. The wider the film latitude, the greater the contrast.
   b. The narrower the film latitude, the lower the contrast.
   c. The wider the film latitude, the lower the contrast.
   d. Latitude and contrast are unrelated.

7. Which film storage considerations can affect the quality of an image?
   a. Temperature
   b. Humidity
   c. Shelf life
   d. All of the above
   e. None of the above

8. Intensifying screens work because of the light photons given off inside the screen by which of the following?
   a. Silver ions
   b. Phosphors
   c. Sensitivity specks
   d. All of the above
   e. None of the above

9. Which statement is true about the use of intensifying screens?
   a. Patient exposure is lower and recorded detail is less.
   b. Patient exposure is higher and recorded detail is more.
   c. Patient exposure is lower and recorded detail is more.
   d. Patient exposure is higher and recorded detail is less.

10. Film cassettes and holders generally have which of the following?
    a. A buffer pad to separate the film and screen
    b. A foam pad to keep the film in contact with the screen
    c. Two different slots into which are slid the film and screen
    d. A plastic divider for positioning the screen at an angle to the film

Key Terms

Before continuing, be sure you can define the following key terms.

Artifact: A mark or image on a radiograph that did not result from attenuation of the x-ray beam as it passed through a patient; it may be caused by heat, humidity, static electricity, damage to the intensifying screen or cassette, mishandling of the film, or other causes.

Atomic silver: A build-up of silver atoms at sensitivity specks as free electrons join with positive silver ions.

Automatic processor: Film developing processor that automatically moves the film through the different stages of developing, fixing, washing, and drying.

Base: The strong layer of film to which the emulsion layers are applied.

Cassettes: Usually made of plastic; holders of film and intensifying screens.

Clearing agent: A chemical in the fixer solution that bonds to unexposed silver halide crystals so that they can be removed from the emulsion.

Contrast: The differences in density on adjacent areas of the radiograph.

Darkroom: A special room where film can be handled outside film cassettes and sealed packages, to be loaded into cassettes, removed from cassettes, and inserted into automatic processors.

Daylight film processing unit: Film processing units not requiring a darkroom; the unit automatically moves film into and out of the cassette, so that handling is unnecessary.

Density: The overall amount of blackening on a radiograph; also called optical density or radiographic density.

Double-emulsion film: Film with an emulsion on both sides of the film base.

Emulsion: The layer in the film that contains the silver halide crystals suspended in gelatin.

Film characteristics: Refers to film speed, latitude, contrast, and recorded detail.

Fixer: The chemical used in the development process that prevents continued exposure of the silver halide crystals and thus "fixes" the visible image.

Fluorescence: A type of luminescence that happens instantaneously with exposure to x-rays and stops when the exposure is terminated; this is the type of luminescence that occurs in intensifying screens.

Grain: The tiny black spots that make up the visible image, one grain coming from each silver halide crystal after exposure and development.

Intensifying screen: A device that converts some x-ray photons to light photons to help create the latent image on the film, thereby reducing the x-ray exposure required.

Latent image: An invisible change in the silver halide crystals of the film's emulsion resulting from exposure to x-ray or light photons.

Latitude: The ability of a film to show different shades of gray, from light to black.

Luminescence: The process by which a material gives off light photons as a result of an interaction with other photons.

Manifest image: The visible image on the film after processing of the latent image.

Phosphor: The crystals in an intensifying screen that emit light when struck by x-ray photons.

Phosphorescence: A type of luminescence that does not stop when the exposure to x-rays is terminated; this type of luminescence is undesirable in intensifying screens.

Recorded detail: The degree of sharpness of structures actually recorded on the radiograph.

Reduction: Part of the development process in which the developer solution neutralizes the positively-charged silver ions in the exposed film crystals.

Replenisher reservoir: Tanks in an automatic processor from which the various chemical baths are refilled or replenished with fresh chemicals.

Safelight: A special light used in darkrooms that does not expose film, so that personnel can see inside the darkroom when film is unprotected.

Sensitivity specks: Impurities in the film emulsion that attract silver ions produced when x-rays interact with the silver halide crystals; these clumps of silver ions are converted into black metallic silver by the development process.

Shelf life: The period of a film's useful life, denoted by the expiration date on the film package.

Silver recovery: A process by which silver in the processing chemicals or unneeded films is captured and recycled.

Speed: A characteristic of a film or intensifying screen, reflecting how quickly it reacts to x-rays; the speed of an intensifying screen refers to how quickly it absorbs x-rays and converts the energy into light photons.

Supercoat: A clear top layer of film that protects the emulsion.

Topical Outline

The following material is covered in this module.

I. Film characteristics vary among different kinds of film for different purposes.
   A. Most films are composed of a base, an emulsion on one or both sides of the base, and covered with a supercoat.
      1. Silver halide crystals are suspended in a gelatin in the emulsion.
      2. The latent image is formed when x-ray photons interact with the emulsion.
         a. Electrons are freed, which migrate to sensitivity specks in the crystals.
         b. Positively-charged silver ions are attracted to the negatively-charged sensitivity specks, creating atomic silver.
         c. The chemical processing converts the atomic silver into grains of black silver.
   B. Specialty films include mammography film, cine film, and duplicating film.
   C. Film characteristics include speed, contrast, latitude, and recorded detail.
      1. Film speed refers to how much blackening occurs as a result of a set exposure.
         a. The size of the crystals in the emulsion is the primary determinant of film speed.
         b. Larger crystals lead to a faster film speed but less resolution because of the larger film grain.
      2. Contrast is the difference in densities on a radiographic image.
         a. High-contrast films have a relatively even grain size, and low-contrast films have more varying crystal sizes.
         b. The choice of a high- or low-contrast film depends on the body areas being imaged and other factors.
      3. Film latitude refers to the range of exposures that can be performed with a film to obtain diagnostically useful densities.
         a. The wider the latitude, the lower contrast.
         b. A film with narrow latitude differentiates more clearly subtle differences in tissue densities.
      4. Recorded detail refers to the extent that small structures can be recorded on a film with sharpness, or high resolution.
         a. The smaller the grain of a film the better the resolution and recorded detail.
         b. Most modern films have such small grain that differences can be seen only if the radiograph is magnified.
II. To prevent problems with radiographs, careful film handling is necessary.
   A. High temperatures can cause fogging on stored film; some departments refrigerate film that will not be used for a while.
   B. High humidity can cause fogging, whereas very low humidity can cause static electricity and potential artifacts.
   C. Any light exposure can cause artifacts or fogging; film should be opened and handled only under a safelight.
   D. Film is very sensitive to radiation, even to scatter from the patient or personnel.
   E. Shelf life is important, and film should not be used beyond its expiration date.
   F. Physical handling must be careful to avoid creasing or bending the film or getting any hand cream or lotion on it.
III. Understanding intensifying screens and film holders is important to obtain good images and prevent artifacts.
   A. The screen is composed of a base layer, a phosphor layer, a reflective layer, and a protective coating.
   B. Fluorescence is the property of phosphor that creates light photons from an interaction with x-ray photons; old screens must be replaced to avoid phosphorescence, which is a delayed light emission.

C. The phosphor crystals are larger than the film crystals and thus reduce image sharpness somewhat; faster screens give off more light photons per x-ray photon.

D. The screen must be in direct, continuous contact with the film; loss of contact causes artifacts in the image.

E. Screens and film holders must be handled carefully, as any damage or warping can cause artifacts.

IV. Film processing involves a number of steps to create the finished radiograph.

A. Daylight film processing units eliminate the need for a darkroom, as the unit loads and unloads film to and from the cassette automatically.

B. Automatic processors carry the film through the cycle of developer, fixer, washing, and drying.

1. A roller transport system moves the film in and out of the baths.

2. Chemicals in the baths are automatically kept at the correct temperature and replenished from separate tanks as needed.

C. The development process makes a manifest image from the latent image.

1. In the developing step, the reducing agent neutralizes the positively-charged silver ions, and visible black specks of silver are converted from the atomic silver.

2. The clearing agent in the fixer removes unexposed silver halide crystals, leaving the manifest image.

3. The wash step dissolves any residual chemicals.

4. The dryer completes the process.

D. Darkrooms are used to load film into cassettes, remove film from cassettes, and load film into the automatic processor.

E. Darkrooms have light-protected entrances and pass boxes for films, using safelights for personnel working inside.

V. Film artifacts may occur from poor film storage conditions, mishandling of film, damaged cassettes or film holders, or problems with the developing process.

VI. Silver recovery is the process of reclaiming silver from processing chemicals and unneeded films, to be recycled.

A. The three types of silver recovery systems are metallic replacement units, electrolytic units, and chemical precipitation units.

B. Unneeded films themselves are stored for recycling.

Review

1. The film emulsion is applied to one or both sides of the film _____, usually made of polyester.

On top of the emulsion is the _____ layer, which protects the emulsion. The emulsion itself is composed of _____ crystals suspended in gelatin. With processing, the exposed crystals, which have been converted into _____,

remain on the film and the _____ are washed away.

2. Film speed depends on the size of the _____ in the film. The larger the crystals, the faster the film, but also the larger the _____ of the image. The _____ of the film depends on the uniformity of the crystals; high-contrast films have relatively even grain size. The choice of what contrast to use in an examination depends mostly on the _____ being imaged. The film's _____ is inversely related to the contrast.

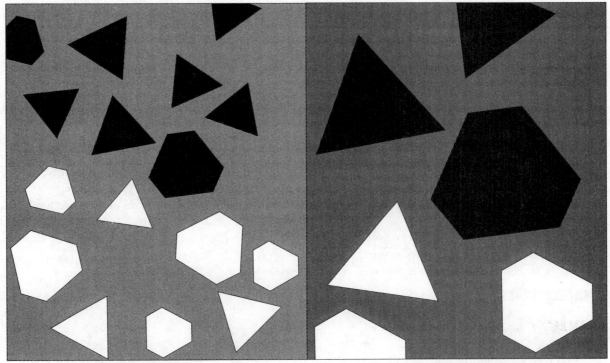

FILM CRYSTALS　　　　　**FILM CRYSTALS**

3. Most films have such fine grain that the human eye cannot detect differences in the amount of _____ in an image unless it is magnified. The crystals of a(n) _____ are larger, however, and therefore there is lower resolution when a screen is used. Screens are used in most exams, however, because of the lower patient _____.

4. Film that is stored at too _____ a temperature may become fogged. Too _____ humidity also can cause fogging, although too little humidity makes sparks caused by static electricity more likely, which can cause artifacts on the radiograph. Because the film is also very easily damaged by exposure to light, it is loaded into film _____ only in a(n) _____. A special light called a(n) _____ inside the darkroom allows personnel to see while they load and unload film.

5. When handling film, take care to avoid getting any _____ onto the film, which may cause artifacts. Also avoid areas of open chemicals, whose _____ can also cause fogging or artifacts.

6. Intensifying screens work because the layer of _____ gives off light photons as a result of interaction with _____. Old screens must be eventually replaced because when the phosphors become exhausted, _____ may occur instead of fluorescence. A screen must be in _____ contact with the film for the best resolution. The _____ the screen, the more light photons it gives off per x-ray photon. One must be careful in handling screens because _____ can result from a bent or warped screen or film holder.

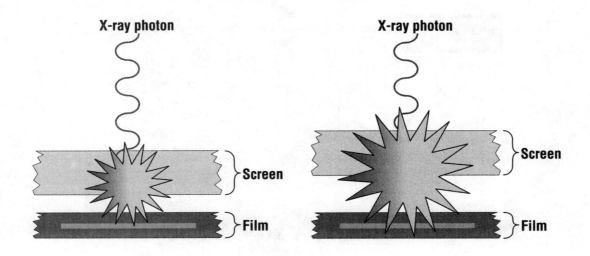

SEPARATION BETWEEN THE SCREEN AND FILM PRODUCES LESS SHARPNESS

7. _____ are used in some departments, which eliminate

the need for a darkroom. Automatic processors handle the processing in most departments, and

have reduced the processing time to about _____. Inside the automatic processor,

_____ move the film from one bath to another and out after drying. The

_____ of all the chemicals is controlled automatically by a thermostat, and

_____ supply additional chemicals as needed.

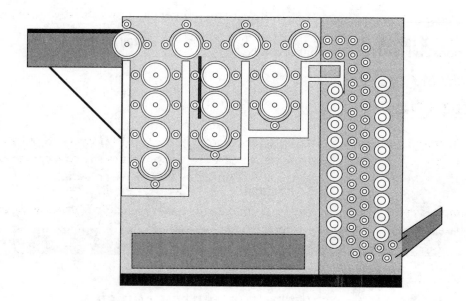

BASIC COMPONENTS OF AUTOMATIC PROCESSOR

8. The first chemical in the process, called the _____, converts the atomic silver into

grains of black metallic silver. In the second chemical bath, the _____ removes the

unexposed silver crystals so that they do not continue to be exposed. The _____ part of

the emulsion is also washed away, leaving the clear film base. The third bath, the

_____, removes any traces of fixer that might turn the image brown or yellow over

time. Then the film is dried.

9. The _____ to darkrooms have been designed to prevent light from entering. Lightproof pass boxes in the wall allow _____ to be brought into the darkroom without letting in light. The room is kept dark except for the _____ light of special safelights that allows personnel to see when handling the film. As with film storage, the darkroom's environment must be carefully controlled, specifically to keep both _____ and _____ within acceptable ranges.

10. _____ is the general term of capturing the silver from the developer solutions and used films, so that it can be _____.

Learning Quiz

The following material includes interactive exercises found in the CD-ROM version of this module operated in the "Student Mode." These questions will allow you to review the concepts presented in this module and will help you gain a more complete understanding of the material.

1. Draw a simple sketch of a cross-section of double-emulsion radiographic film, showing and labeling the film base, the emulsion, and the supercoat.

2. Describe what happens in the formation of the latent image on the film after exposure to x-rays. Then describe what happens during film development that converts the latent image into a manifest image.

3. Explain the trade-off that occurs with film speed. What is the big advantage of faster films? What is the disadvantage?

4. List as many factors as you can think of that should be controlled during film storage and handling. (List 7 to 10 items.)

5. Explain why an intensifying screen must be positioned immediately next to the film.

6. Below is a sketch of the inside of an automatic film processor. Draw lines to the following key parts and label them:

Developer solution
Fixer solution
Bath
Dryer
Film entrance slot
Film exit slot
Transport roller

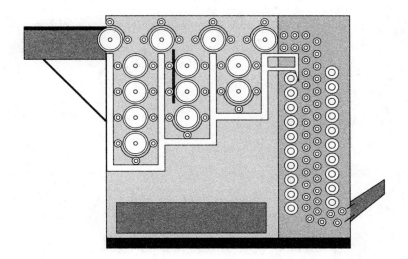

BASIC COMPONENTS OF AUTOMATIC PROCESSOR

7. What are the three primary uses of the darkroom?

List other things you would typically find in a darkroom.

8. List as many causes of artifacts as you can.

Applications

1. Explain what is different in the silver halide crystals of high- and low-contrast films. Give at least two examples of types of exams that show when a high-contrast film and a low-contrast film would be used.

2. Just as there are high- and low-contrast films as well as different film speeds, intensifying screens also vary in speed because of phosphor crystals of different sizes. Explain why most departments use standard film-screen combinations rather than each being selected individually for an examination.

3. Explain what could happen to an image if a film cassette is warped and in one section does not provide good contact between the film and the intensifying screen. How might that section of the image look?

Posttest

Circle the best answer for each of the following questions. Your instructor has the correct answers.

1. The silver halide crystals in the film emulsion are suspended in a gelatin that allows which of the following?
   a. Exposed crystals to remain on the film
   b. Unexposed crystals to wash away during development
   c. The film base to remain clear
   d. All of the above
   e. None of the above

2. What is needed to convert a latent image into a manifest image?
   a. Expose the film
   b. Develop the film
   c. Place the film in a viewbox
   d. All of the above
   e. None of the above

3. What happens when photons interact with silver halide crystals in the film emulsion?
   a. Electrons are freed in the crystal.
   b. Electrons move to sensitivity specks.
   c. Sensitivity specks gain a negative charge.
   d. All of the above are true.
   e. None of the above is true.

4. Atomic silver results from the joining of which of the following?
   a. Silver halide crystals with sensitivity specks
   b. Silver ions with the film developer
   c. Free elections at the sensitivity speck with silver ions
   d. None of the above

5. With most modern films, which affects sharpness more?
   a. The size of the film crystals
   b. The size of the intensifying screen crystals
   c. The composition of the film/screen cassette
   d. All affect sharpness equally

6. Film storage temperatures that are too high could cause which of the following?
   a. Fogging
   b. Slowing of film speed
   c. Breakdown of the film base
   d. All of the above
   e. None of the above

7. Light photons given off by the phosphors in an intensifying screen travel in what direction?
   a. In all directions
   b. Toward the reflective layer, then toward the film
   c. Directly toward the film
   d. Depends on whether a grid is used

8. An intensifying screen may produce a poor image if it is which of the following?
   a. Dirty
   b. Scratched
   c. Warped
   d. All of the above
   e. None of the above

9. Modern automatic processes develop the film to a final stage in what amount of time?
   a. 5 to 10 minutes
   b. 3 to 5 minutes
   c. 1 to 3 minutes
   d. About 1 minute or less

10. Rollers inside an automatic film processor are used to do which of the following?
    a. Move the film through different chemical baths
    b. Transport the chemicals to the film in stages
    c. Evenly spread each chemical over the surface of the film
    d. Fix the image in the emulsion by applying pressure

11. What is the first chemical bath in the automatic processor?
    a. Fixer
    b. Developer
    c. Wash
    d. None of the above

12. The fixer does what in the development process?
    a. Removes unexposed silver halide crystals from the emulsion
    b. "Glues" the metallic silver to the film base
    c. Turns the atomic silver into black silver
    d. Turns the film base clear

13. What is the third step in the development process?
    a. Developer
    b. Fixer
    c. Wash
    d. Drying

14. Which variables should be controlled in the darkroom?
    a. Temperature, humidity, light
    b. Light
    c. Temperature, light, and sound
    d. Light and temperature

15. What is a type of silver recovery system?
    a. Metallic replacement unit
    b. Electrolytic unit
    c. Chemical precipitation unit
    d. All of the above
    e. None of the above

Answer Key

Answers to Pretest

1. c

2. a

3. c

4. c

5. a

6. c

7. d

8. b

9. a

10. b

Answers to Review

1. Base, supercoat, silver halide, black metallic silver, unexposed crystals

2. Crystals, grain, contrast, body part (or tissue), latitude

3. Recorded detail, intensifying screen, dose

4. High (or warm), high, cassettes (or holders), darkroom, safelight

5. Hand lotion, fumes

6. Phosphors, x-ray photons, phosphorescence, direct, faster, artifacts

7. Daylight film processing units, 90 seconds or under 1 minute, rollers, temperature, replenishment reservoirs

8. Developer (or reducing agent), fixer (or clearing agent, or hypo), gelatin, wash

9. Entrances, cassettes (or film), red, temperature, humidity

10. Silver recovery, recycled

Answers to Learning Quiz

1. Your sketch should show the base in the middle, a layer of emulsion on both sides of it, and a supercoat layer as an outer layer on both sides.

2. When film is exposed to x-rays, some x-ray photons strike some film crystals. This causes electrons in those crystals to be freed, and they migrate to the sensitivity specks in the crystals. These specks then have a negative charge, which attracts positive silver ions. This build-up of silver ions at the sensitivity specks is called atomic silver. It makes the latent image, which cannot be seen.

   In the development process, the atomic silver is converted into black metallic silver. Each exposed crystal becomes one black grain. The unexposed crystals are washed away. Therefore the manifest image is formed of black silver grains on the clear film base.

3. The advantage of faster film speeds is that shorter exposures can be used to make the image. With fast films, more blackening occurs more quickly, requiring fewer x-ray photons to make the image. This occurs because the silver halide crystals in fast films are larger, and fewer crystals need to interact with x-rays in order to form the image. And that is why there is a trade-off: fewer large crystals also means the image is composed of larger grain, or is said to be grainier. With most modern films this is an issue only if the film is magnified, because the human eye cannot see the grain otherwise.

4. Factors to control during film storage and handling include the following:

   Temperature
   Humidity
   Light
   Radiation
   Shelf life
   Storage position
   Bending, scratching
   Marring with hand creams or lotions
   Chemical fumes
   Correct placement in undamaged cassette or holder

5. An intensifying screen must be placed immediately next to the film to minimize the distance light photons travel from the phosphor crystals to the film crystals. Remember that the light photons generated from the interaction with x-ray photons will be moving in all directions. Those on the film side may spread out slightly before reaching the film, and those moving in the other direction reach the reflective layer and then bounce back to the film, also possibly spreading out slightly more before reaching the film crystals. This spreading out of the light photons that will make the image means the resolution is not quite as good when a screen is used. The closer the phosphor layer is to the film emulsion, the less spreading there will be and the better the resolution. Any perceptible distance between the screen and the film will significantly diminish the quality of the image.

6. Compare your labeling to that shown here:

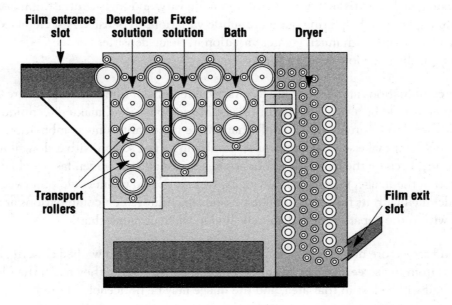

BASIC COMPONENTS OF AUTOMATIC PROCESSOR

7. The three primary uses of the darkroom are as follows:
   - To load films from packages into cassettes
   - To remove exposed films from cassettes
   - To insert exposed films into the automatic processor

   Other things you would typically find in a darkroom include stored film, chemicals for processing, a silver recovery unit, a safelight, counters for work space, and lightproof film pass boxes in the wall.

8. Artifacts may be caused by any of the following:

   High temperature (in storage or processing)
   High humidity
   Static electricity caused by low humidity
   Exposure of film to light
   Exposure of film to radiation
   Scratches or marring of the film
   Scratches or marring of the screen or film cassette
   Exposure of film to chemical fumes
   Hand lotion or other substance on the film
   Damaged or warped cassette causing poor contact of screen and film
   Film used beyond its expiration date

Answers for Applications

1. High-contrast films, which show very few shades of gray, are composed of silver halide crystals of relatively even size. In the emulsion of low-contrast films the crystals vary in size, giving a wider range of response and more shades of gray.

   High-contrast films are used when tissue densities in the body area being examined have a small range. For example, breast tissue has less variation in density, and high-contrast film is usually used in mammography to help bring out more subtle variations in density. A skeletal examination, on the other hand, with much greater variation in tissue densities between bone and soft tissues, would typically use a low-contrast film.

2. Film-screen combinations are used mostly for practical reasons. If film and screen were selected separately, there would be a much larger list of possible combinations, making technique charts very unwieldy with too many possibilities. Perhaps more important, some combinations might result that would not make sense. For example, combining a fast screen with a slow film would have little value, because the larger phosphor crystals that make the screen fast would determine the resolution of the image, making it more grainy even if the slow film could otherwise have been more detailed with its fine crystals. The best possible film-screen combinations are generally worked out within the department and are reflected in the technique charts.

3. If the film and screen are not in good contact in one area because of a warped cassette, then the light photons from the screen will spread out more in that area before they reach the film. Recorded detail will be lost in that area, and the image may be noticeably blurred.

Notes

Notes

Notes

Notes

Notes

Notes

Notes

Notes